Academic Life
AS SEEN BY OTHERS

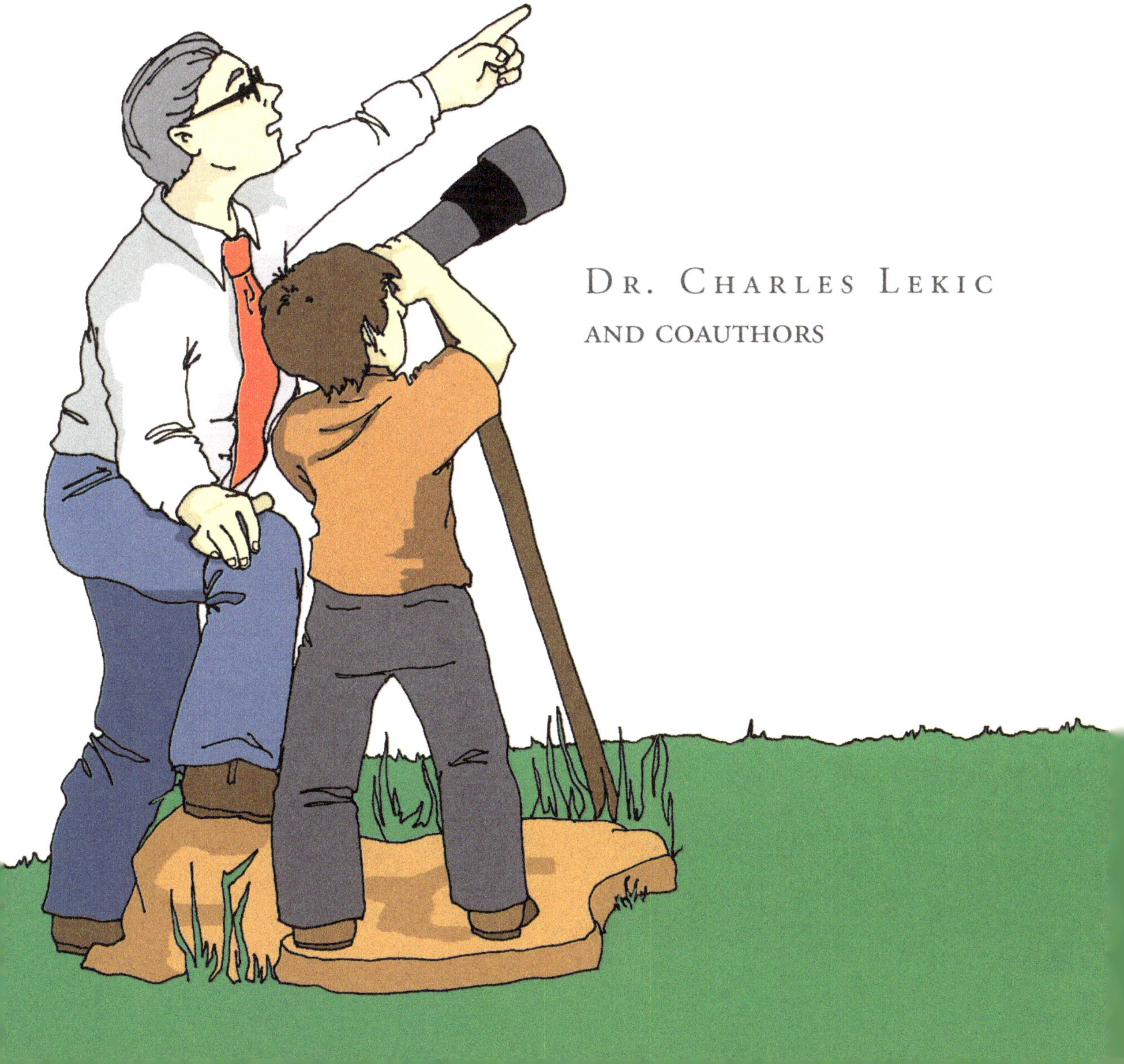

Dr. Charles Lekic
and coauthors

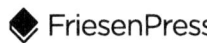

Suite 300 - 990 Fort St
Victoria, BC, V8V 3K2
Canada

www.friesenpress.com

Copyright © 2017 Dr. Chalres Lekic
First Edition — 2017

Cover and interior illustrations art by Shannon Parish
Book deisgn by: Rebecca Finkel, F + P Graphic Design

All rights reserved.

No part of this book may be reproduced or transmitted in any form by any means,
except for brief excerpts used in a review, without prior written permission from the copyright holder,
which may be requested through the publisher.

ISBN 978-1-5255-1651-1 (Hardcover)
978-1-5255-1652-8 (Paperback)
978-1-5255-1653-5 (eBook)

1. MEDICAL, DENTISTRY

Distributed to the trade by The Ingram Book Company

Dearest Val,

You are my most favourite dental assistant I ever worked with!

With best wishes
Charles

Contents

Why an academic? 7

Preface 9

Part One 13

Caring 15
    Dr. George Loewen 15
    Claire Common 17
    Hamish Varshney 19
    Mike Botsford 20
    Samer Mudher 21
    "The Pedo Class" 23
    Brett Luschinski 24
    Deb Adleman 25
    Ryan Head 27
    Sunayna Gupta 29
    Elena Ferrer, Class of 2011 31
    Dr. Ryan Cormack, Class of 2011 33

Gratefulness 35
    Anis Sabet 35
    Kunit Nagra 36
    Shima Gharib 37
    By a pediatric dentist, ... 39
    Eric Kristof, Class of 2001 41
    Dr. Christina Chan 43
    Fadi Kass, Class of 2002 45
    Julie Maniate 47
    Robert Pesun 49
    Mark Berscheid 51

Teaching 53
    Darci Bonar, Class of 2011 53
    Omar Mohammad, ... 55
    Alex Serebnitski 57
    Jay Biber 58
    Harpreet Sroay 59
    Jennifer Coutu 61
    Kiranpal Kaur Sroay 62
    Amanda Huminicki 63
    Cameron Grant 68
    Anonymous 71
    Edina Heder 73
    Sherif Elsaraj, Dent 2010 Class President . . . 75

Part Two 77

Working with less than 10 years 79
    Diane Mymko 79
    Val Friesen 80
    Adriana Salles 81
    Debbie Saunders 83
    Tony Iacopino 87

Working with between 10 and 20 years 89
    Sandra Dufour 89
    Leona Vos 91

Working over 20 years 93
    Robert Diamond 93
    Howard Cross 95
    Billy Wiltshire 103

Summary 104

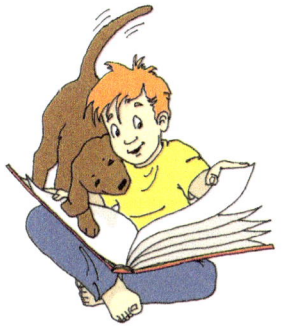

Turn the page please

Why an academic?

Becoming an academic may involve many different reasons and those reasons often change over the course of a career. If one reason is to be the only remaining one, it will be the joy of having the purpose in life. In academia we all learn to better ourselves as well as to become all we can and to discover our potential.

I could agree with that.
Charles Lekic

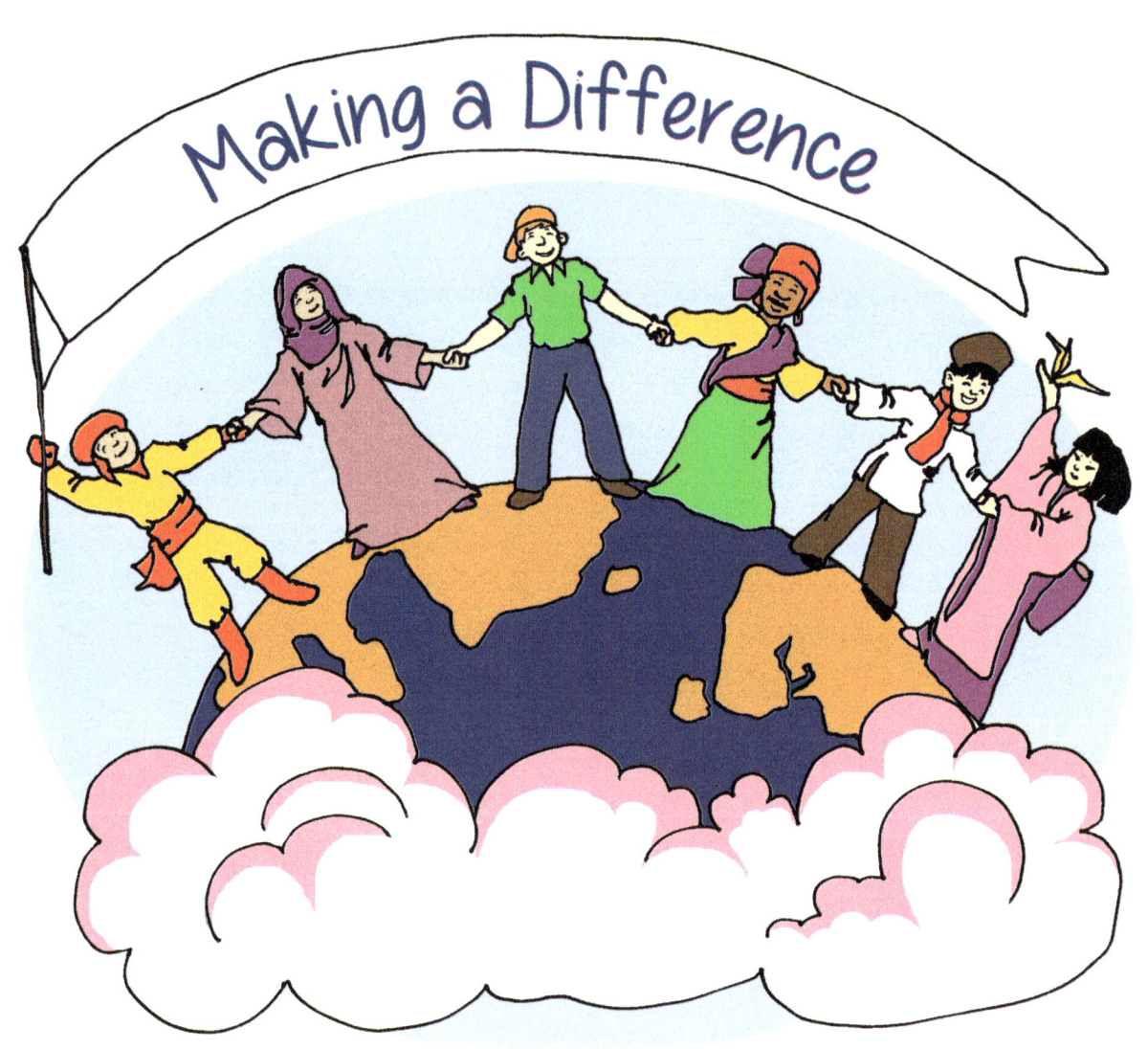

Preface

A FEW DECADES AGO an extraordinary individual declared, "I have a dream ..." With those words my life's idol was born. For it is after every dream that a new day starts, a new vision can arise, and new directions can be followed. A great amount of research has been done in an effort to improve our understanding and interpretation of dreams, but for modern science dreams are still a mystery. Outside of science, there exist many individual interpretations of how dreams relate to both past and future events. In those interpretations some dreamers are certain "that they have already seen events and the things in their dreams." Expectations that dreams may help us improve the understanding of the future are the reason why sometimes dreams and more often "big dreams" may be the call to follow this dream and make it happen. For those dreamers certain they have seen a future worth having, the decisions they make today will be ones to make that dream happen.

It was more than 30 years ago that I woke up one morning excited about a dream. In that dream I had become a teacher. Now at that point in my life, I was a young dental graduate with "big plans", but in reality had no real plan. Today, I am not sure that I can recall the exact details of the dream, but I do remember how excited and overwhelmed I was to have the opportunity to live the dream of becoming a teacher/academic. This dream would allow me to make a difference in the lives of others and give back to the future members of our profession gifts I had received from my own teachers not long before. At the same time, I started challenging the dream. I recalled occasions when as a dental student I had experienced difficult times, especially when the teaching process would unnecessarily use the "big stick policy". (For those of you unfamiliar with the term, the "big stick policy" is a style of teaching that uses fear of consequence to motivate action.) That famous phrase, "I have a dream …", changed the world, and it helped me to understand the importance of living my own dream. A dream to try and contribute to changes that one day would see the "big stick policy" in education forever walk into the history books.

I have lived this teaching dream at a handful of universities during my academic career. The longest and most recent part of this dream was at the University of Manitoba and lasted 20 years. I remember well my first year in Winnipeg and the stories of the challenges the students were experiencing. It is important to hear these stories and to share some of your own challenges – not only to make ourselves feel better, but to the desperation we felt and to see that future generations of professionals would not have to experience the same. From that first year onward, I had a number of meetings with students. The most important changes I made to the undergraduate program and the start-up of the graduate program happened because of the valuable comments and suggestions I received from them.

Living the academic life was an incredible dream, and I do not regret a day of it. Certainly not because of the salary, or the meetings – most of which I disliked, or the University rules – many of which I wonder why they even exist. No, the reason I do not regret a day of my academic life is because of the overwhelming feeling of accomplishment one has seeing students dramatically improve and move forward in a relatively short period of time. Using the words of a dreamer, it is like a little bird that cannot walk when entering school and after few years can now "spread its wings and fly" to provide great care to their future patients.

In pediatric dentistry we always tried to teach with a "no big stick policy." Interestingly enough, a number of students went on to enroll in pediatric dentistry graduate programs, and today Winnipeg has one of the largest numbers of pediatric dentists per capita in the country. Perhaps my dream of contributing to the "no big stick policy" has been achieved? This is a question that, when answered only by the academics, would be very selfish indeed. To truly come to this conclusion, it is necessary for the recipients of the education to let us know if this has been their experience or not. To this end, the graduates, residents, and staff from the University of Manitoba were invited to write about their memories and experiences of working with me during my 20 years there. In doing so, I hoped it would be a potentially valuable testament to what the academic life has meant to those partaking in the teaching process. It would also help me understand if my life really had made the difference I dreamed it would, or else perhaps reveal what I could have done differently to be more successful. To ensure an honest account, a promise was given to every contributor that no changes would be made to the original text and that the text would be included whether signed or anonymous. It was also understood that in my role as author, after receiving their text, I would have the liberty to write any comments I might have in the Summary section of this book.

Collectively, as students and teacher, contributors and author, this book has sought to reflect on an academic life as viewed by others. Together we hope to try and bring more light on this life and the dream that guided it. We trust that in doing so it will inspire and help future generations of professionals decide if this too could be a dream worth following – the academic life.

Thank you and hope you will enjoy the book!
—Charles Lekic

PART ONE

Caring

Gratefulness

Teaching

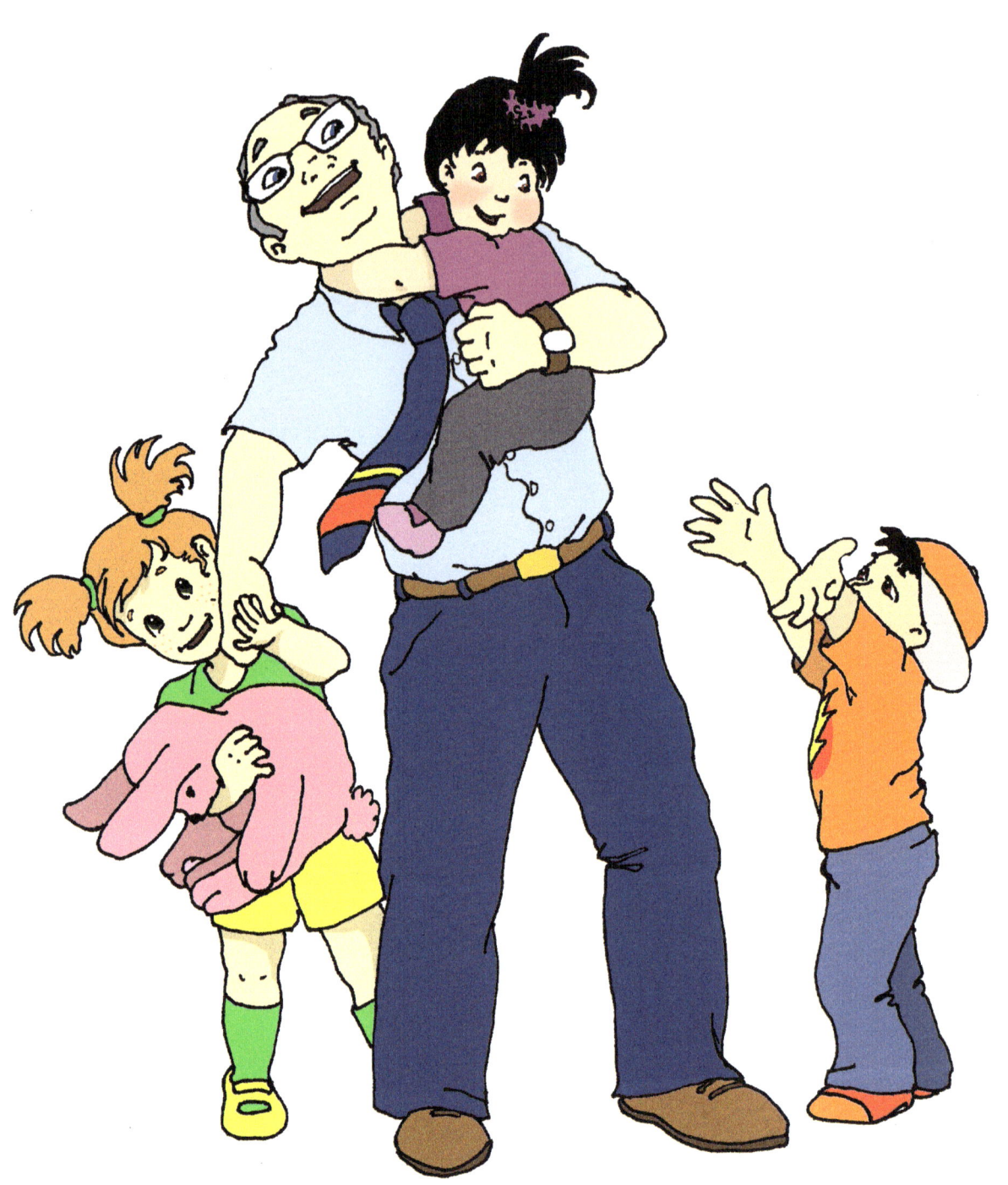

Happiness is . . . Working with children.

Caring

Laughter is the best medicine

My first experience with Dr. Lekic was before dental school while shadowing him at Children's dental world. I had a very positive experience watching him entertain and interact with children, almost as if there was no needle involved in dentistry. Dr. Lekic was very charismatic with patients, family, and staff. His silly jokes with children made everyone laugh and created an environment that was fun for the child. The experience with Dr. Lekic had completely convinced me that dentistry was a great career choice.

Almost three years passed before actually becoming an official student of Dr. Lekic during second year dentistry, pediatrics. Much of those times were pre-clinical and thus listening to him lecture. My greatest memory of him during that time was the passion, enthusiasm, and most importantly his humour and ability to make everyone smile during his lectures. Sitting for his lectures was a pleasure and something I would look forward to listen to him speak.

During the next two years of third and fourth year of dentistry was more patient involvement and less time lecturing. We covered the same information booklet/notes given to us in second year, but it would be more clinical application and board exam based. I would remember that sparse time lecturing became more precious and valuable; every word that came from him was a word of wisdom. Clinical memories composed of a very busy pediatric clinic on Fridays with plenty of patients, with lots of help from the pediatric residents. Fridays were a day to look forward to.

It has been a pleasure to be part of Dr. Charles Lekic's legacy.
—Dr. George Loewen

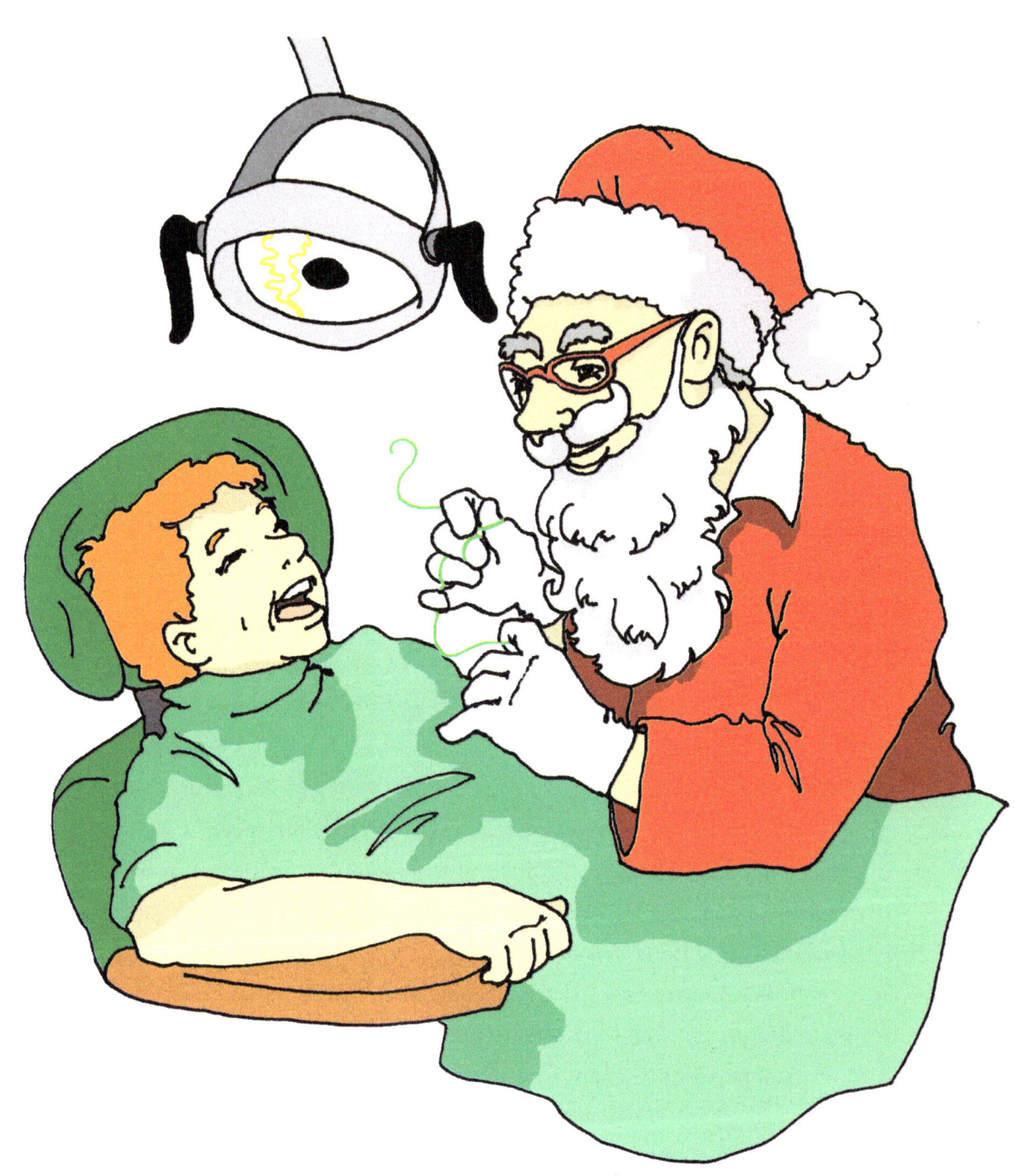

Here comes Santa floss.

I remember Fridays at the faculty well.
Looking on the board to see if you were in one of the back "quiet" rooms, which meant that your kid might give you some challenges, and then the anticipation of the bus arriving to meet whoever you were going to treat. Dr. Lekic was always there with a smile on his face, greeting the kids as they came through the door. The most fun times were on special occasions like Halloween or Christmas when Dr. Lekic would be dressed up as a clown or Santa Claus, causing so much excitement with the kids within the clinic. In the first dental school I attended, I didn't get much experience treating children, and Dr. Lekic really opened my eyes to the fact that it can be good fun and very rewarding to win a child's trust. I now quite enjoy having children come into my office and the laughs that they give us.

—Claire Common

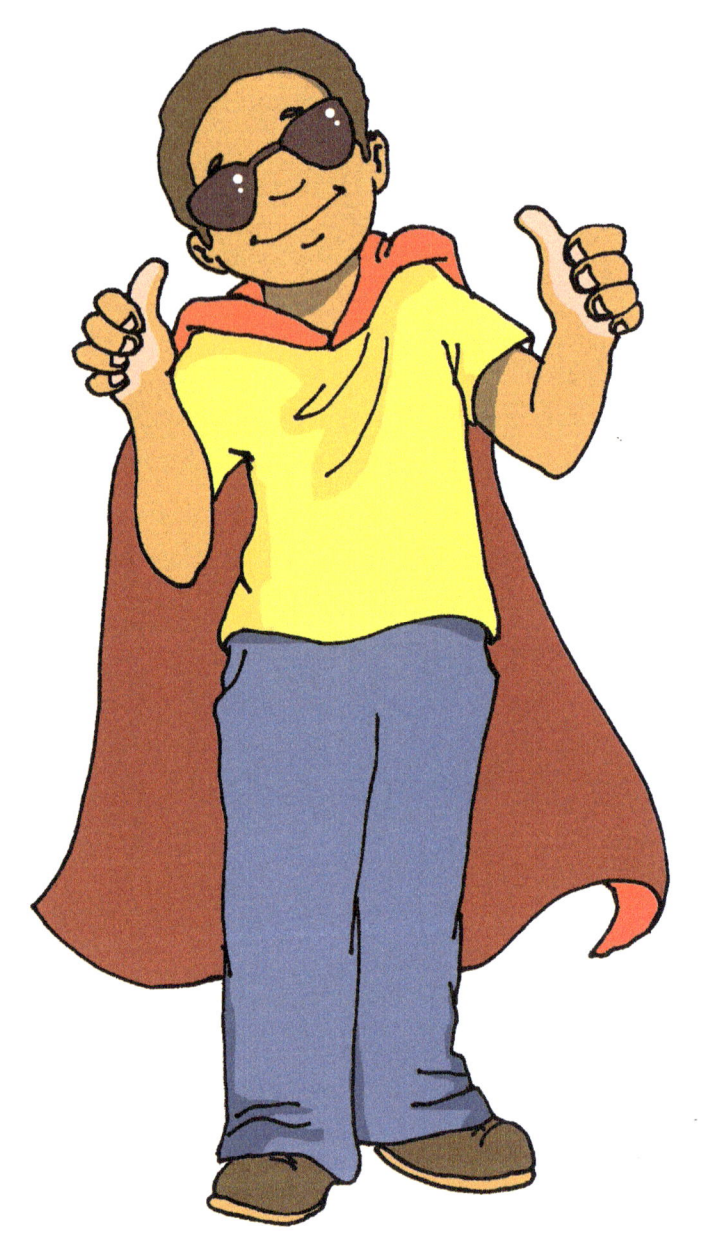

Cool guy!

Hi Dr. Lekic,

I do have something to share with you (about you) ...

At the University of Manitoba (Faculty of Dentistry), you were one of the kindest professors there. There is one memory I have of you that always makes me smile ... and it has nothing to do with dentistry!

One day, after clinic, I was walking out of the Brody Centre (atrium). I was crossing the street at a four-way intersection. Anyways, this car starts to go through, even though I had the right of way. I was about to yell at the driver when I looked in the windshield and saw that it was Dr Lekic! Instead of him yelling back, he gave this huge grin, and his face lit up in a way that was kind and apologetic. At that point I just smiled and waved back. Dr Lekic somehow took a potentially negative situation, and, through a power he has, turned it into a positive and happy outcome. Only Dr. Lekic could do that.

Thanks for everything, Dr. Lekic. You are the best!

Yours truly,
—Hamish Varshney

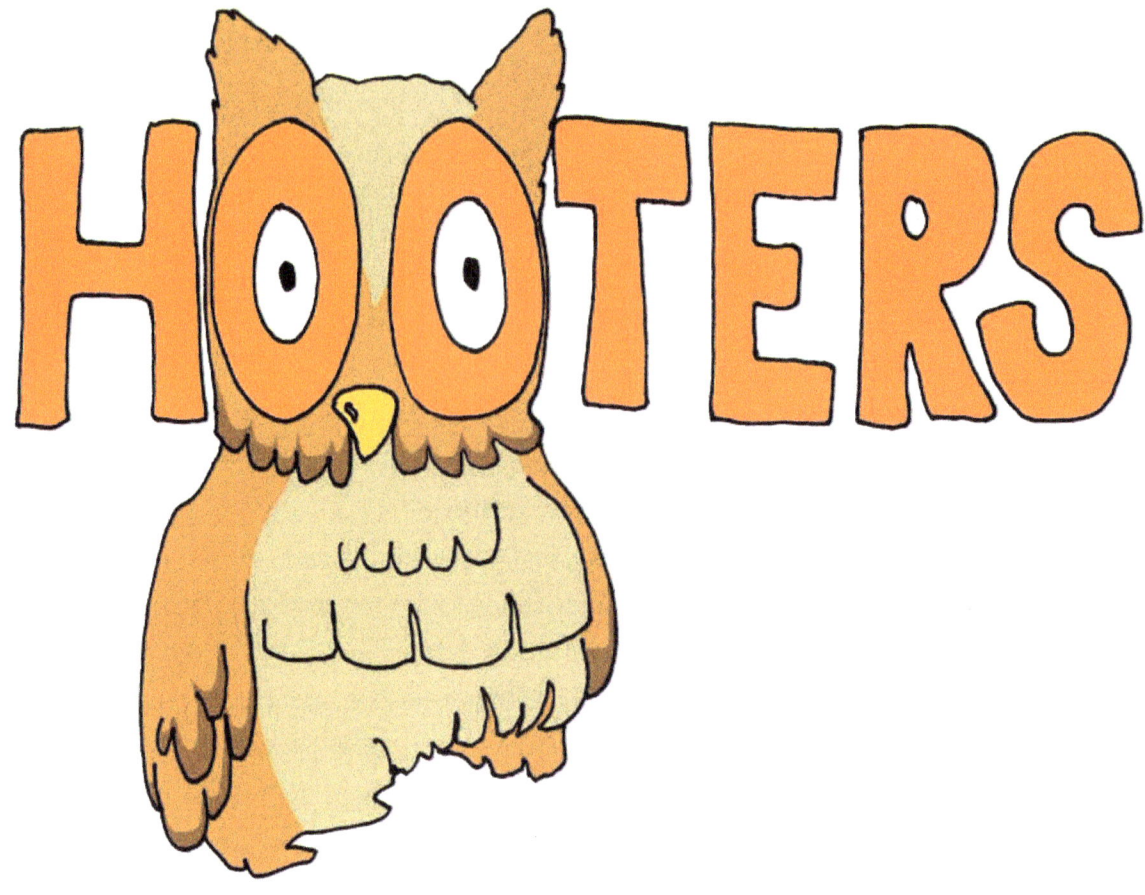

Fridays on the clinic floor.

Ortho and Pedo in a laid-back learning environment – can't get any better, right? Unless your prof offers to take you and some of your classmates for lunch, then lets you drive his new Jaguar! This was repeated the next year, but the restaurant was different (Hooters) and the car was a new Audi.

—Mike Botsford

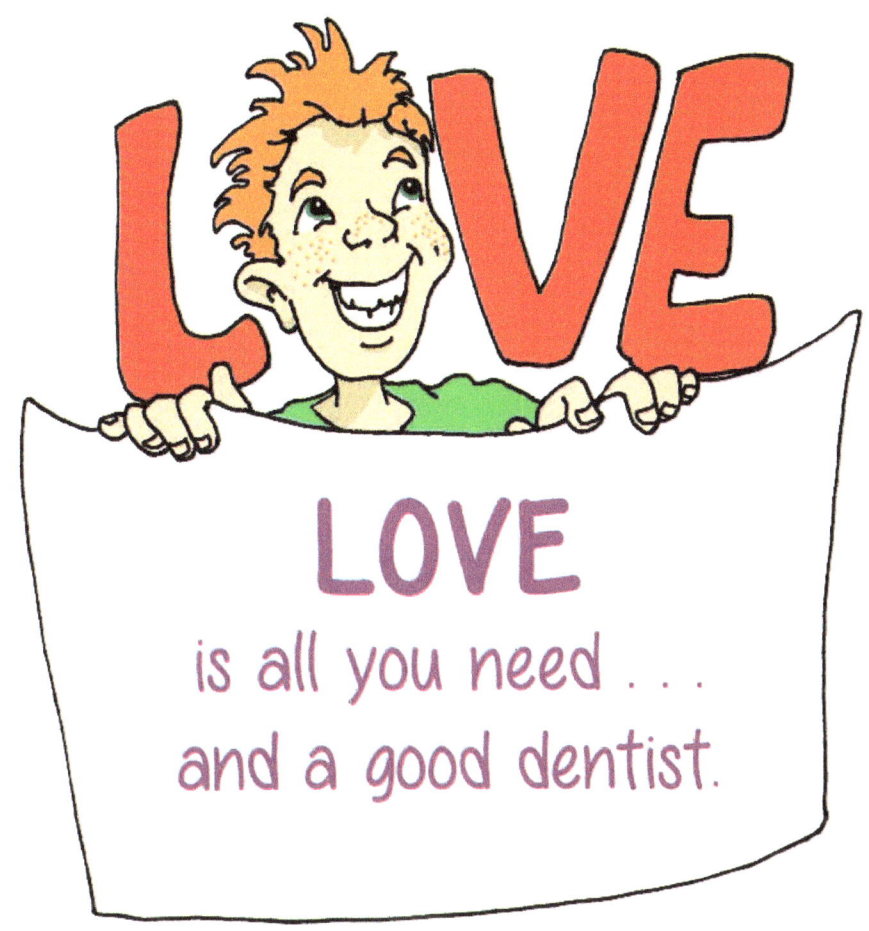

Hi Dr. Lekic,

Thanks for having us for that wonderful dinner, and I hope you will enjoy this new chapter in your life :-)

Personally, I always remember you with your positive and encouraging attitude; professionally, as a mentor and a teacher, you taught us a lot in Dentistry, but more importantly, you taught us the art of caring for our patients because that is who you are: a caring father, teacher, and great person.

Cheers,
—Samer Mudher

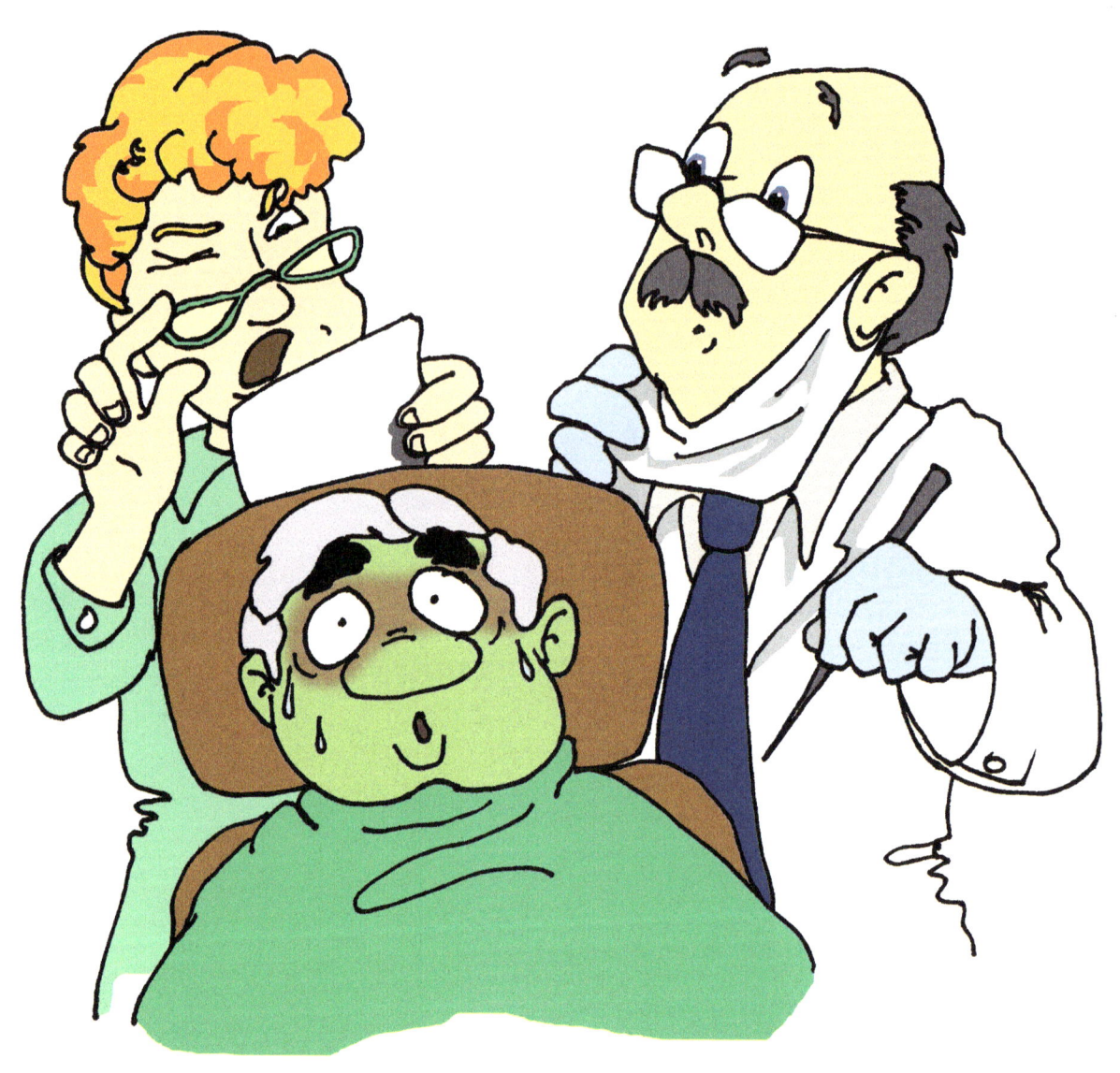

Uhhh, let's see . . . plague . . . plaq . . . Oh, PLAQUE!

Presented to Dr. Charles Lekic

> *Teacher* – realizing that if you stop growing today, you stop teaching tomorrow.
>
> *Educator* – searching out the way people learn to determine how to best teach them.
>
> *Activator* – maximum learning is always the result of maximum involvement.
>
> *Communicator* – real imparting of information requires the building of bridges.
>
> *Heart-impacting Passion* – teaching that truly impacts is not head to head, but heart to heart.
>
> *Encourager* – teaching is most substantive when the learner is properly motivated.
>
> *Readiness* – teaching-learning process is most effective when both teacher and student are adequately prepared.
>
> (taken from *Teaching to Change Lives,* Howard Hendricks)

Thank you for transforming us into caring and technically-competent dental professionals. We deeply appreciate the passion for dentistry that you have infused into all of us as our teacher and mentor. It is our hope that we can pay forward your teaching to future generations of dentists.

From
"The Pedo Class"
University of Manitoba Facility of Dentistry
Class of 2002

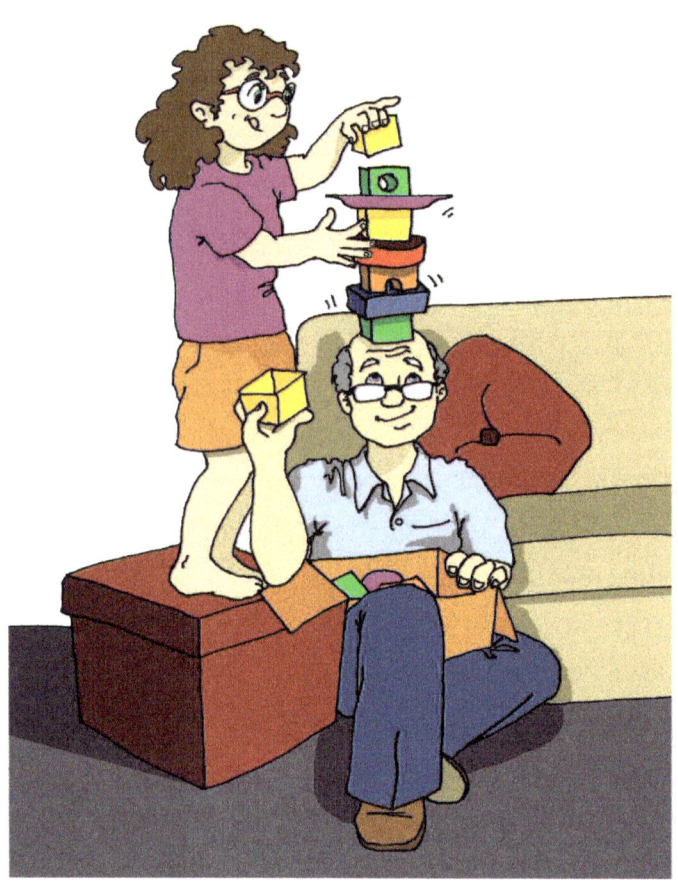

The most valuable thing you can give someone is your time.

Thanks Charles for supporting me through my struggle and stress of dental school. I was targeted for being myself. I felt alone and depressed to be at school. Your inspiration and confidence to be yourself has inspired me to be a great practitioner. Patients love my honesty and candour. I feel like your support through the difficulties and stresses has led me to be the best person possible in the community. Rather than a shying away or conforming to a mold, I have stood out and been more successful for that reason. Thanks for letting me be me.

Thanks,
Brett Luschinski

P.S. Also thanks for letting us wear pink scrubs in clinic.

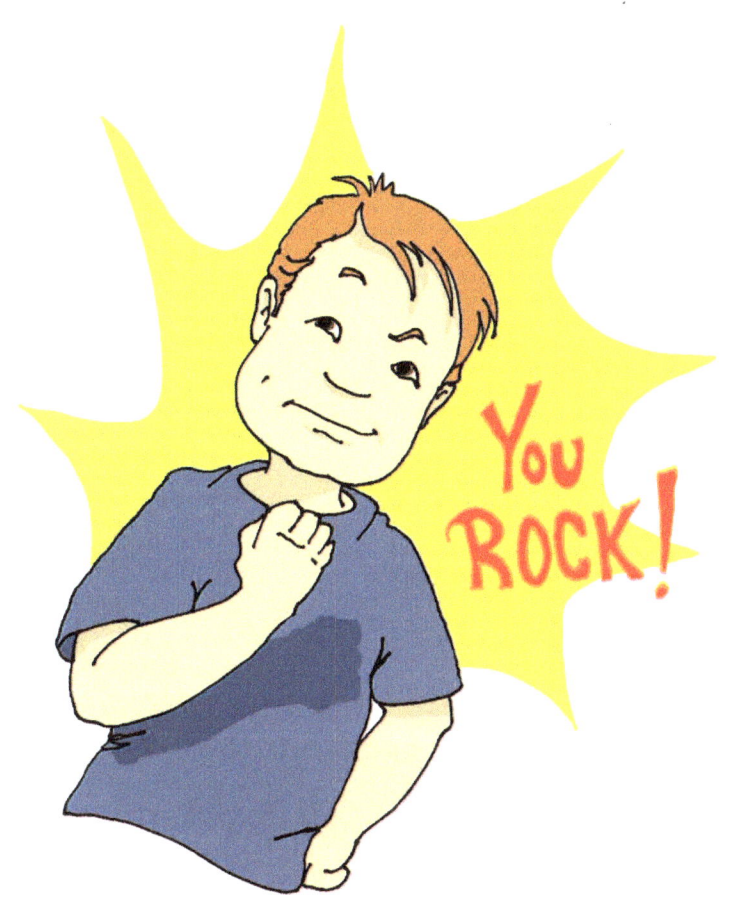

Dear Dr. Lekic,

Special people like you make the world a brighter place. Congratulations on a well-deserved retirement! Thank you for the mentorship, kindness, and respect you offered me through the years of dental school. You were truly a gift to myself and so many.

Sincerely,
Deb Adleman

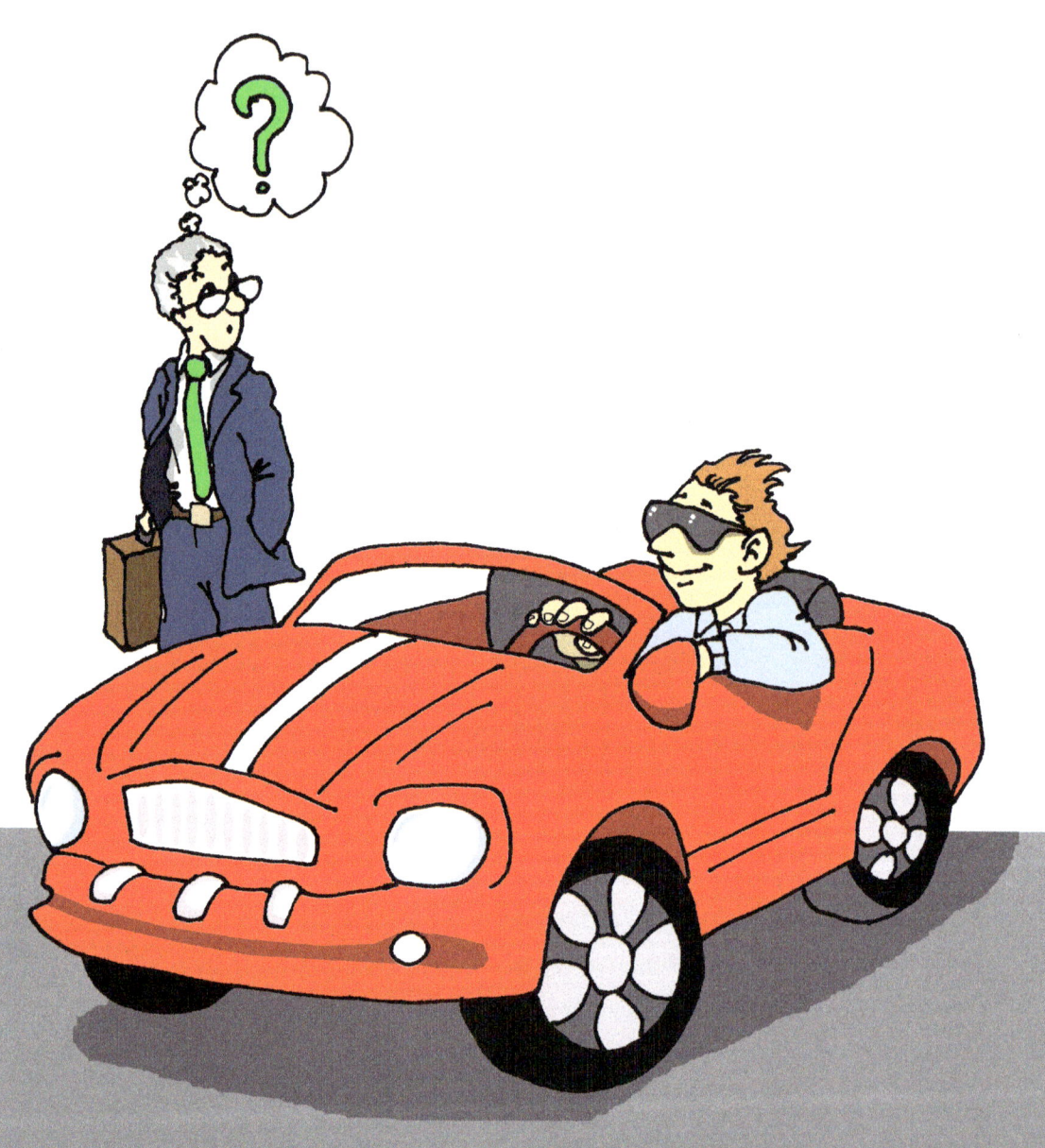

Sorry your students drive nicer cars than you.

Dear Charles,

Thank you very much for inviting me to your retirement party. It was great to see everyone and celebrate with you on your special day. I find life gets very busy, and it is hard to find the time to sit down with friends and colleagues and reminisce of all the good and bad that had transpired over the years. Your retirement party was an excellent opportunity for me to catch up with friends and celebrate your next adventure in life.

    I also want to take this opportunity to thank you for being exceptionally kind and caring to me. From when we first met in first year dental school until today, you have always been very approachable and compassionate towards all of your students, and it shows by the support people gave you during your retirement party. I really enjoyed seeing your passion for both dentistry and cars. I will always appreciate the conversations we have had about both of these topics. I remember you welcoming my class of 2010 into your home on numerous occasions and taking the time to get to know each and every individual student. It has been a pleasure to get to know you over the years, Charles.

> I wish you all the best in your retirement,
> RYAN HEAD

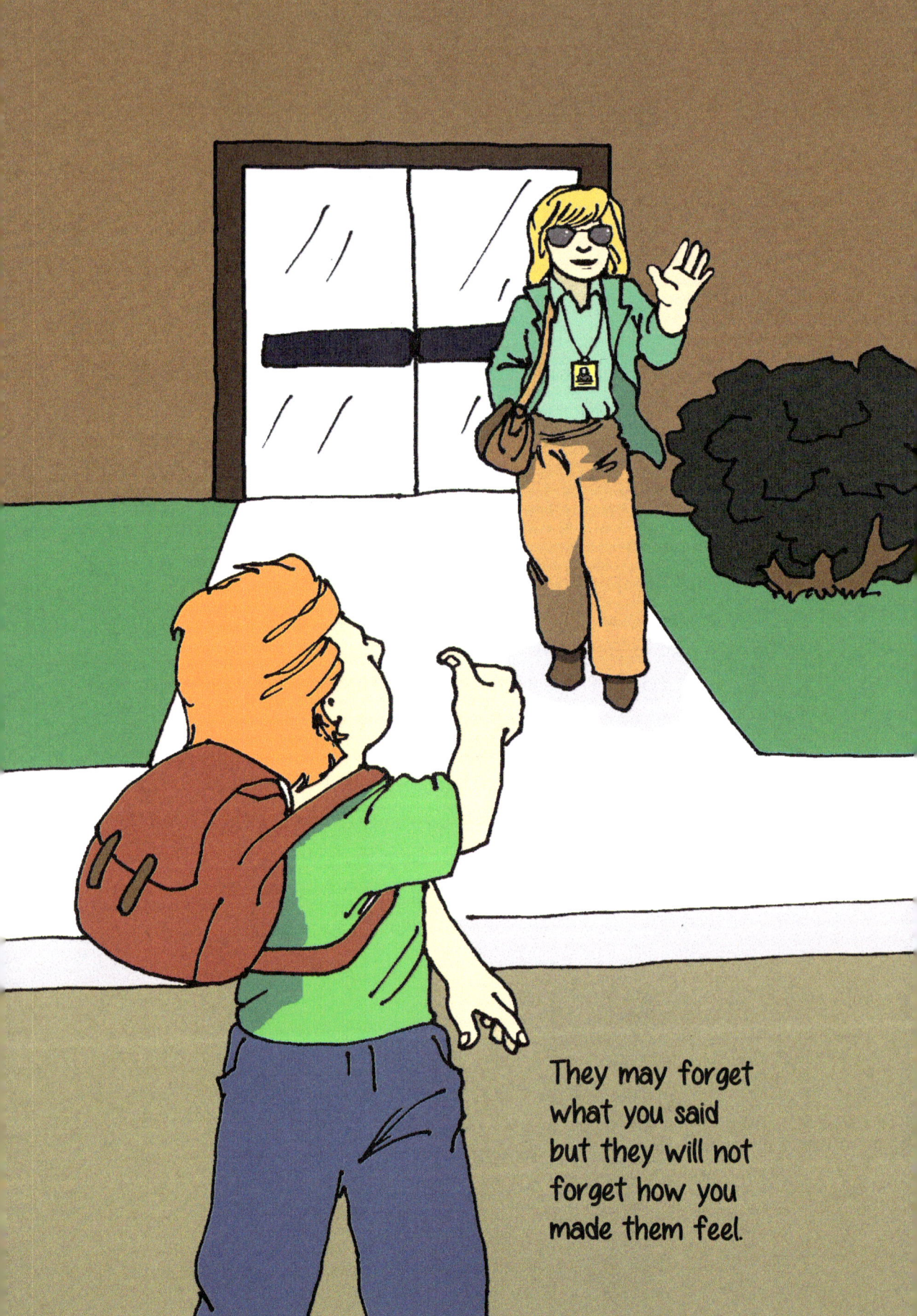

Dental school can definitely be overwhelming. It is a demanding curriculum, and it is very easy to feel lost at times. Fortunately for my class, we had Dr. Lekic as our class advisor. Dr. Lekic emphasized something (and continued to do so) during our four years of dental school that no *one* else really did – caring. He said it every time we saw him. In fact, he placed so much emphasis on it, he even implemented "caring awards", where we would nominate fellow classmates for various acts of kindness. He explained that caring is imperative in becoming a successful classmate, dental professional, and human being. That resonated with me immensely. Now, as a friend, wife, mother, and dentist for almost five years, I remember Dr. Lekic's words almost daily. Thank you, Dr. Lekic, I will always be grateful.

Thanks again,
Sunayna Gupta

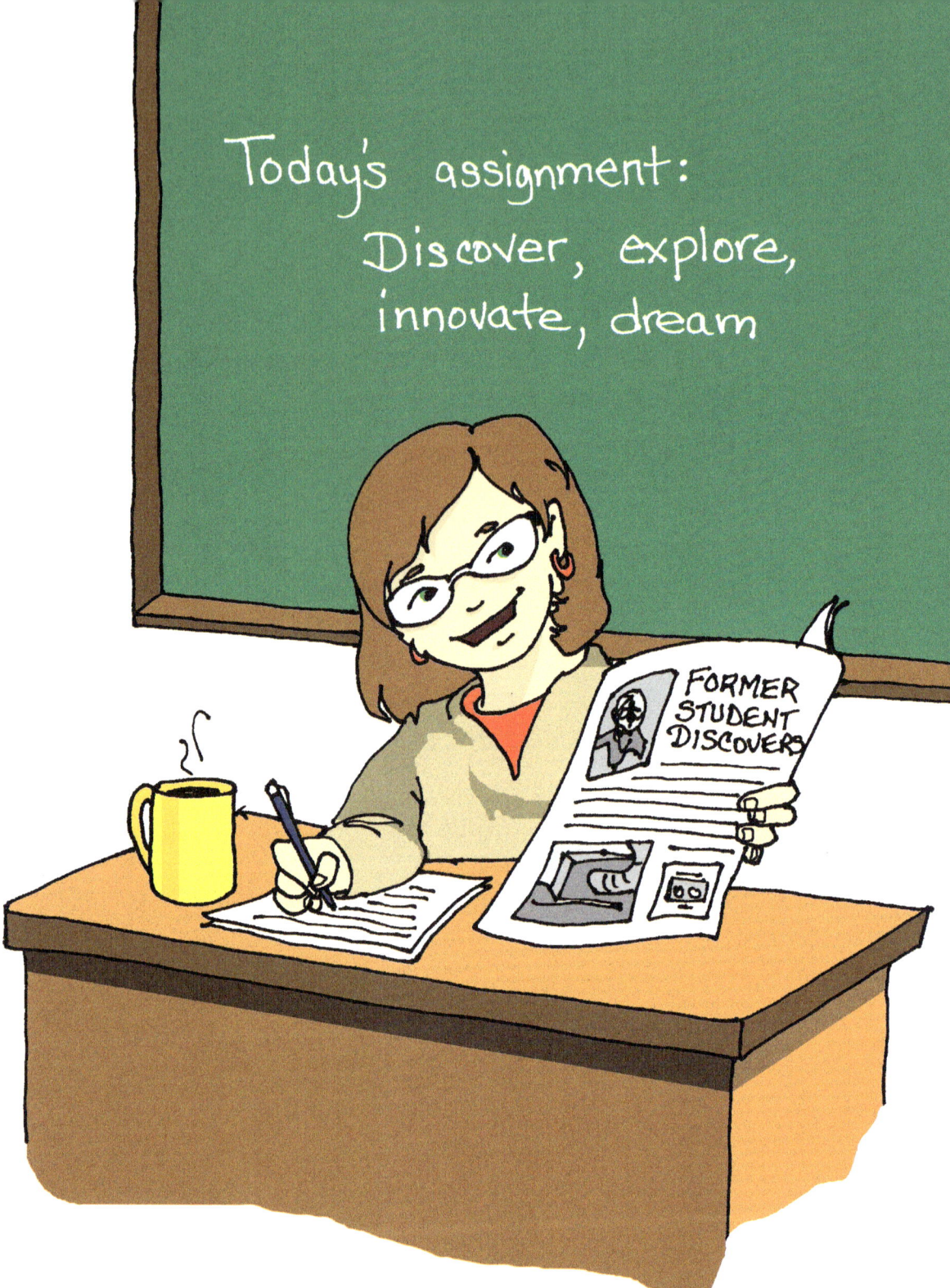

I care more about the people my students become than the scores on the tests they take.

I had the pleasure of having Dr. Lekic as both my class advisor and instructor. Dr. Lekic made it very clear that in order to be the very best dentist you could be, you needed one essential characteristic: to be caring at all times. He didn't lecture on making sure your preparations were perfect or your fillings were contoured just right, but rather that each patient be treated as if they were your own dear family. I have held on to this notion ever since I set foot into the dental clinic.

In a world where clinicians are at times thought to never make mistakes and to be perfect at all times, it is very easy to have unrealistic expectations of ourselves.

Dr. Lekic's lesson provided me with a realistic and attainable goal to reach and strive for each day. It has helped guide me in being the very best clinician I can be, and for that I will be forever grateful to him.

—Elena Ferrer, Class of 2011

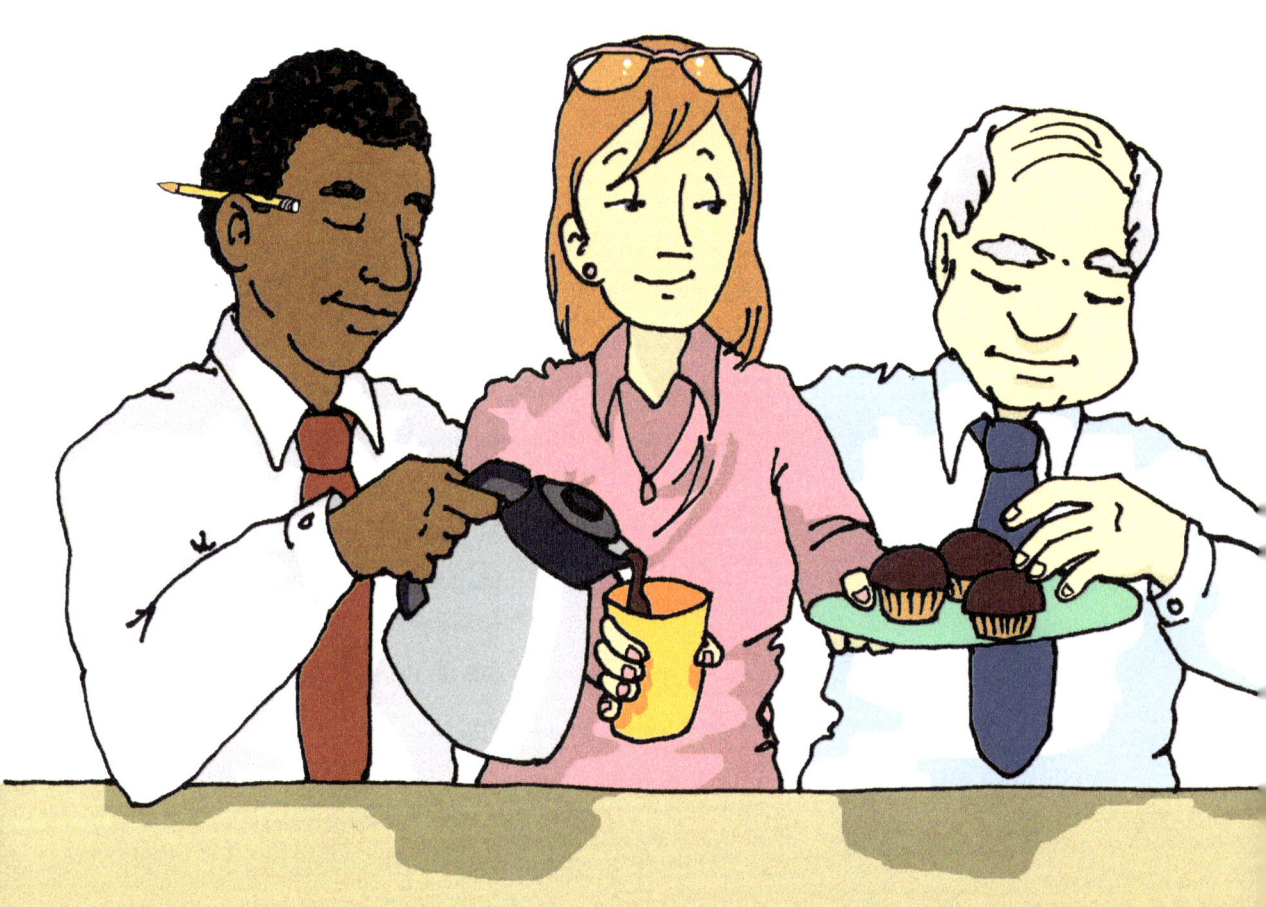

Good people bring out the good in other people.

I have a great deal of respect for Dr. Lekic and his style of leadership and teaching. He was our class advisor during the four years of dental school. From the very first meeting to the last meeting we had with Dr. Lekic, his message and mantra was always about caring: caring for the patients, caring for each other, caring for the instructors. At our monthly meetings, he would hand out "caring awards" based on nominations he received from others in the class. His emphasis on caring helped unify our class and helped us to succeed both individually and as a team.

Dr. Lekic went out of his way to help us with our concerns and requests for change and improvement. He also wasn't afraid to take a stand and tell us "no" on rare occasions when our requests were a little unreasonable. These rare moments reinforced in my mind that it wasn't about popularity or appeasement, but he was authentic and sincere about his passion for being caring to everyone.

Dr. Lekic also expressed his gratitude on a frequent basis. I can recall how full of gratitude he was when we gave him a Santa suit as a gift. He was so happy, I thought he would burst. Moreover, at our monthly meetings we had with him, he would frequently express his gratitude to us for caring for each other and would share his specific observations of our caring he personally witnessed. Even when he was having terrible back pain, he was expressing gratitude.

Dr. Lekic led by example. He knew that a teacher and a leader who genuinely cares, encourages the best in others, and expresses gratitude often will have a significant, positive influence in the lives of his students and followers. I'm grateful for his example.

Sincerely,

Dr. Ryan Cormack, Class of 2011

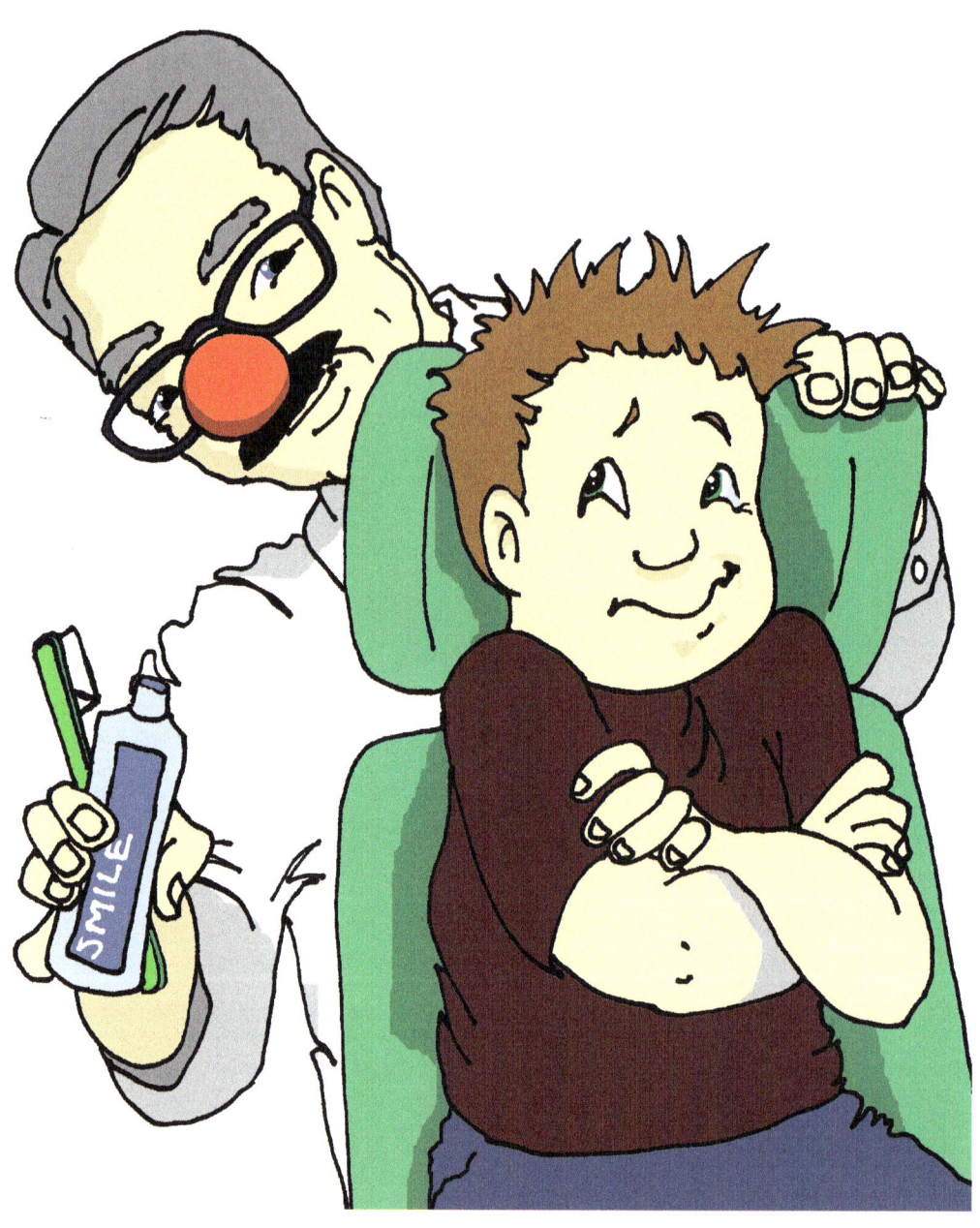

I love people who can make me laugh,
when I don't even want to smile.

*G*RATEFULNESS

Dear Dr. Lekic,

I wanted to write you a note to mention how grateful I am to have had you as a professor, advisor, example, and friend. Your constant joy and hopefulness of your work and patients has inspired me greatly. Regretfully, I was unable to make it to your retirement party. I truly felt humbled to have been even invited to celebrate your time at the university and the exemplary path of service you carved for us all in the profession.

Your unbounded joy allowed me to imagine my work with a lens of possibilities. Your open heart and love for people moved me to see my patients as brothers and sisters, and to view my work as complete, selfless service to them. Your example of coherence between being a father, husband, and a high-level professional allowed me to see that everything is possible if we are just happy.

My words cannot adequately describe how grateful I am for our time together. Thank you so very much!

—A*nis* S*abet*

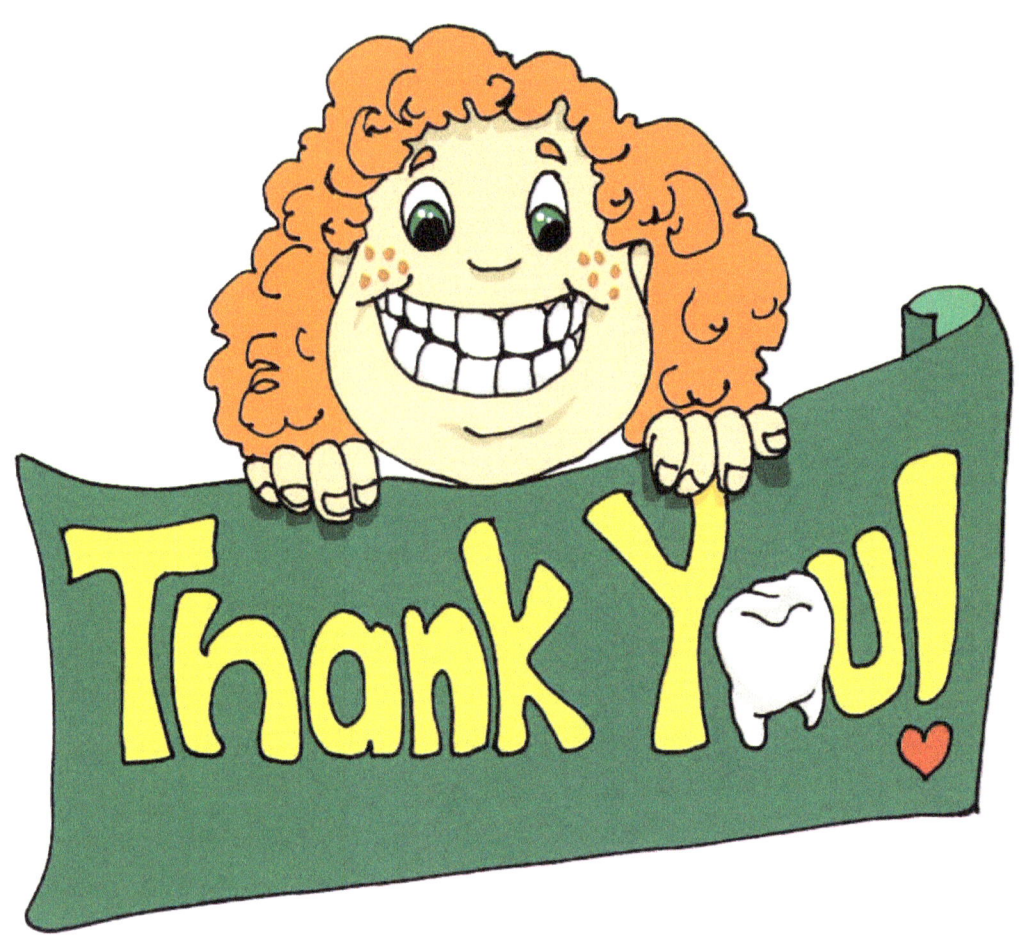

Hi Dr. Lekic,

From the first time I met you, I have always seen you as an advisor, mentor, and father. I cannot thank you enough for all the support you have been giving me for these past 10 years now ... I would not be where I am today if it wasn't for you. Thank you for everything!

—Kunit Nagra

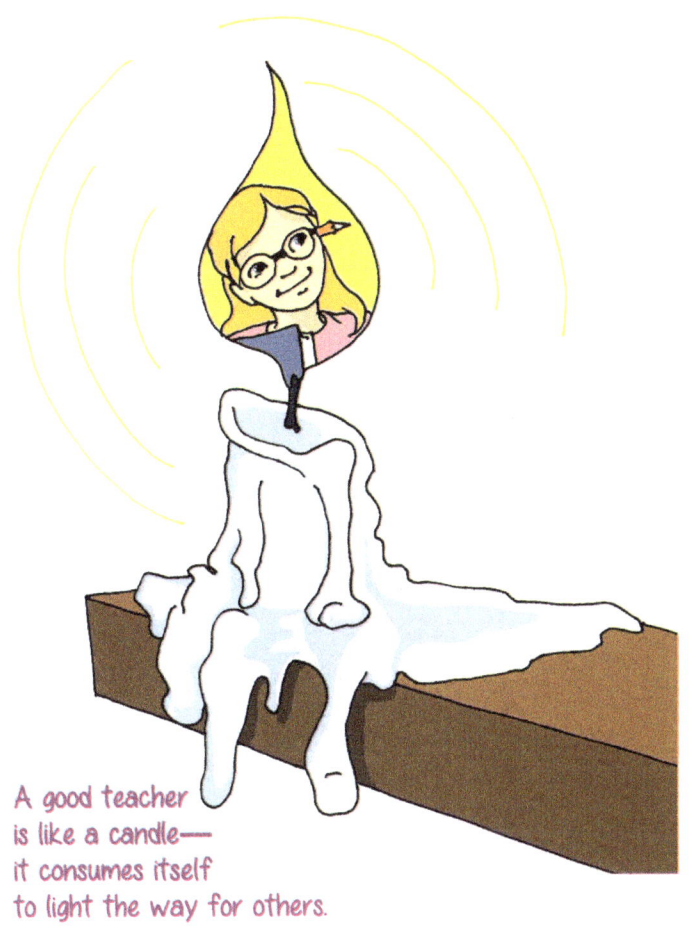

A good teacher is like a candle—
it consumes itself
to light the way for others.

When I was third year dental student and mentioned to Charles I'm interested to become a pediatric dentist one day, he suggested I should apply for pediatric dental internship first to improve my résumé to make a stronger candidate and also to get a better understanding of what a pediatric dentist do. We both looked at the schools offering these internships and realized UofT deadline to apply was just the day after. Dr. Lekic wrote a letter of reference for me the very same day; he even offered to mail it for me with Expresspost! Something no one else would ever do or offer to do on such a short notice! He is the most student advocate person I have ever seen in my whole life! I'm very sad he is leaving, but I wish him all the best.

—Shima Gharib

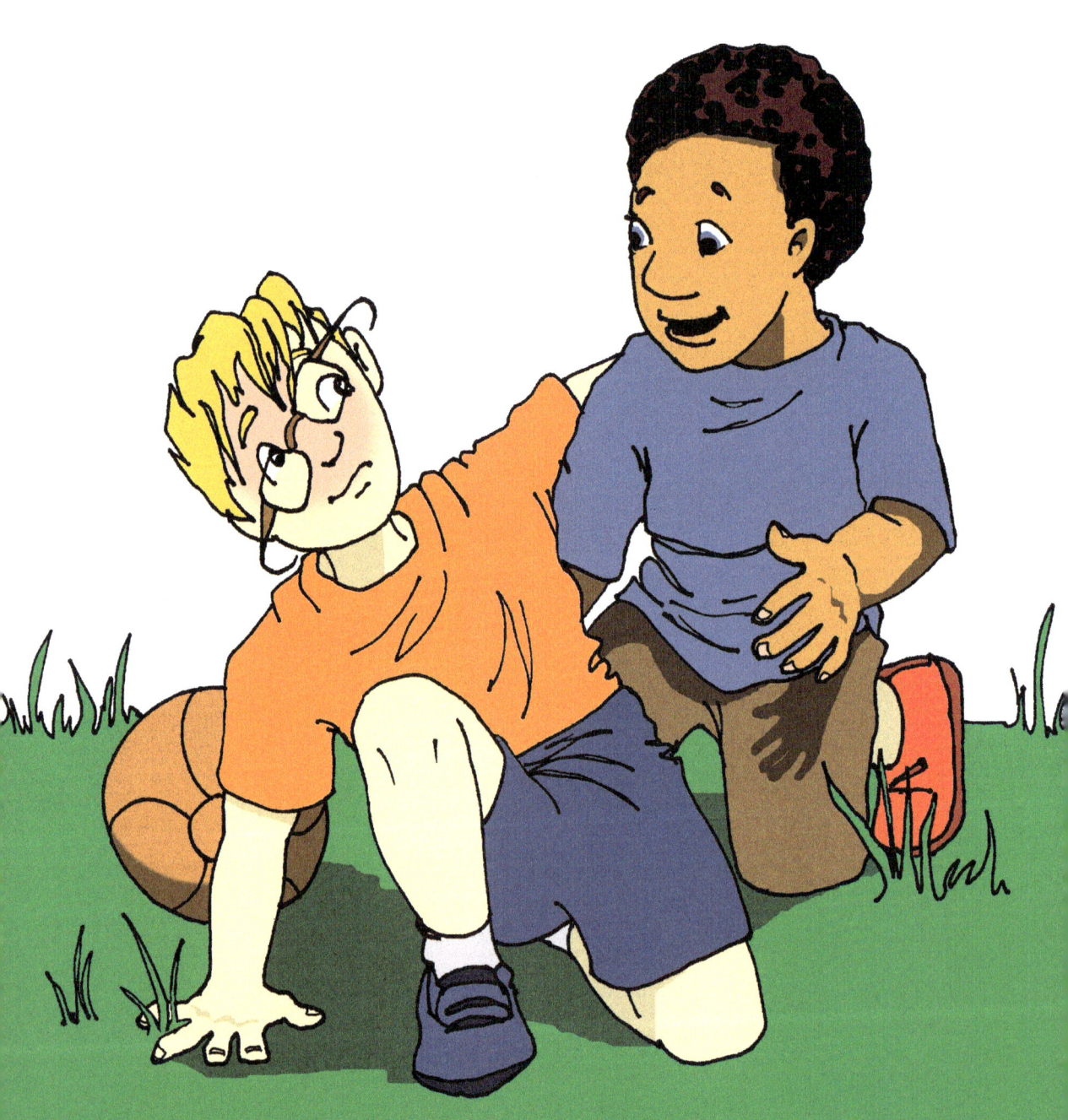

My Grandpa says if you do your best
no matter what the score . . . you win!

This is a story about why I became a pediatric dentist. It happened while I was in third year dental school. It was the beginning of the year, and at that time I did not have much clinical experience with patients. This particular day was a "pedo" day, where we see exclusively young children in the clinic. I was assigned a three-year-old boy to do an examination as part of my slate for the day. This particular child was very active. So active in fact, his mother had to put him on a body leash. At the time I had never seen a body leash before and presumed that the child was autistic or somewhere along that spectrum. Now that I am older and a father of three, I realize that the child was very likely normal and was just high energy. In fact, I also own one of those body leashes and see its benefits in keeping my kids out of trouble.

As I was assigned to do an examination on this child, I made an attempt to look at this child's teeth. Unfortunately, due to lack of skills, I failed miserably. I then went over to the supervising pediatric dentist, who happened to be Charles Lekic, for assistance. He came over and worked what appeared to be magic and did an examination on the child. It was at this time that it became evident that this child needed extensive dental treatment, including crowns, extractions, and fillings, all under general anesthetic. The mother was in quite a lot of distress hearing this as she did not have the financial means to afford the recommended care. Unfortunately, this is quite common in the profession, as children with low socio-economic status are much more likely to have dental disease. Dr. Lekic was very understanding when talking with the mother. He ensured her that he would make sure that the dental work would not cost her anything. In addition, although there would be a cost for the general anesthetic, he would do his best to get that waived as well. The mother was quite relieved and thankful, and the look of relief on her face was extremely memorable. This act of altruism by Dr. Lekic touched me in such a way that I wanted to be a pediatric dentist as well. To this day I am very thankful of my experience and inspiration, and I work and strive to live up to the high standard of being in this noble profession of pediatric dentistry.

—By a pediatric dentist,
a servant of the community and an ever thankful former student

Note: I would appreciate it if my share of any proceeds for the sale of the book be donated to your favorite children's charity.

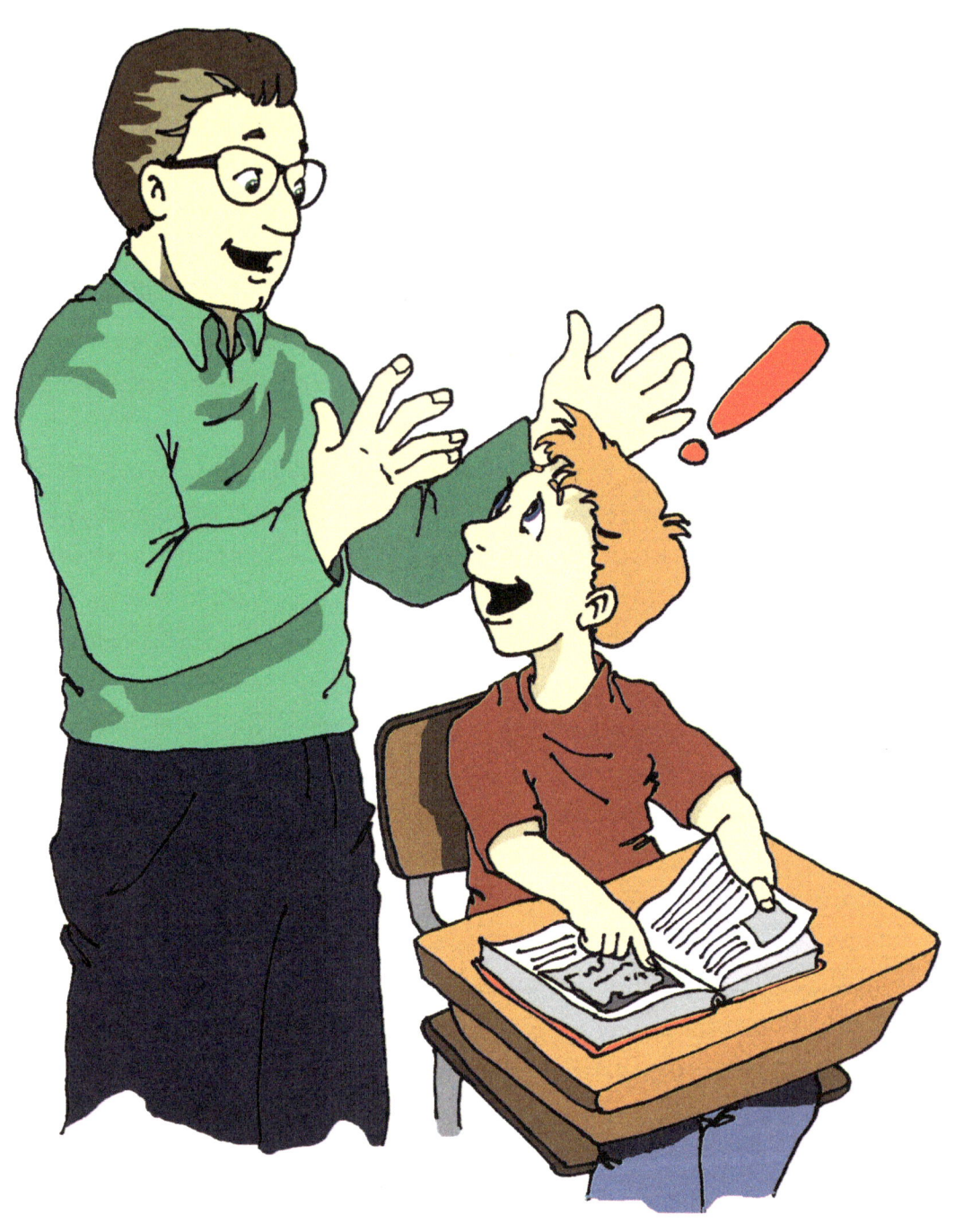

A good education can change anyone.
A good teacher can change everything.

Out of all of our subjects we needed to study in dental school, I felt that we were the most prepared for the real world in pediatric dentistry. This was all done without making any of us feel afraid of our instructors, which was not unusual for all the other dental subjects.

We were not afraid to have a normal conversation with Dr. Lekic, ask him out for lunch (to places we would never consider going to with any other instructor), or even ask him to drive his car (because it was so nice). He has touched our lives in such a great way; I do not think we will ever forget the great learning experiences we have been given or how much we appreciated everything he has done.

—Eric Kristof, Class of 2001

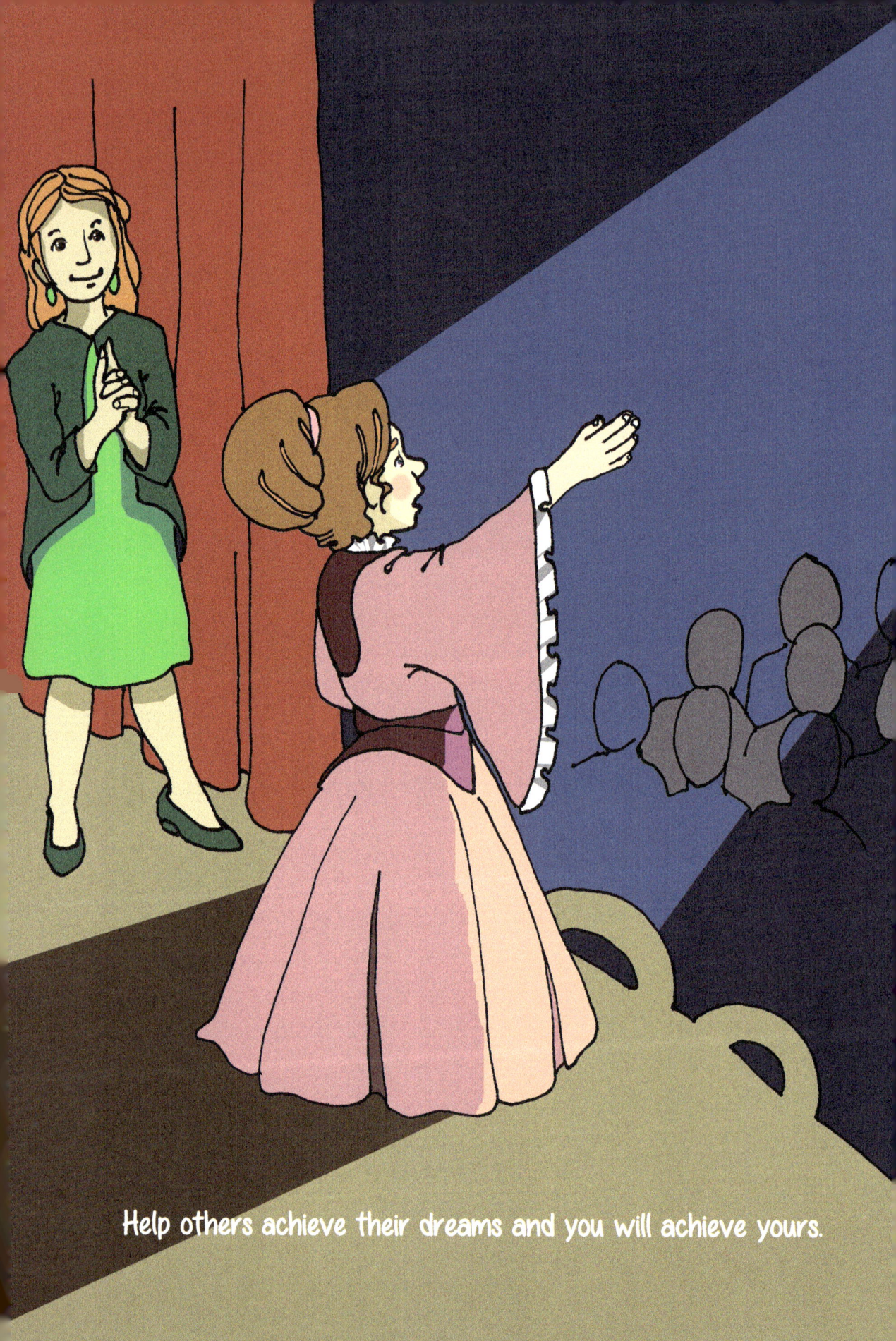
Help others achieve their dreams and you will achieve yours.

Dr. Charles Lekic is one of the most influential teachers I will probably ever have in my life. Charles truly made an impression on me when I found him in a hospital bed with severe back pain but still working on the accreditation for the graduate pediatric dentistry program. I have never met any academic as dedicated to his students and teachings as Charles. He never give himself an excuse not to be better. He always tried to achieve his utmost best for his students – to teach them and to protect them. This was the main reason I applied to the graduate pediatric program at the University of Manitoba. Because I know I can learn to become the best possible version of myself from Charles and I know that he will never give up on the program and what he promised his students – "to teach them to become better than himself." He did not only teach me to become a successful pediatric dentist, but also how to be a caring and responsible individual. I truly owe my successes to him.

—Dr. Christina Chan

My first lecture with Dr. Lekic was indeed a memorable one.

Pediatric dentistry, unlike other disciplines, does not start till the latter part of the second year of dental school. By that time the students had met most of the professors, and the ones who had not personally instructed us, well, their personalities were down to rumours handed down from senior students. And the rumours about Dr. Lekic were simple: he was the 'nicest guy' to ever teach. Well, I was about to experience this first hand.

It had been a long week, busy, and I had a few late nights studying and perhaps enjoying the life of a carefree student a bit more than I'd like to admit. So in I went to Dr. Lekic's first ever lecture. In his usual manner, his style of lecturing was very entertaining and most of us were absorbed. However, in the second part he dimmed the light so we could better see the slides that he was projecting. Sitting in the back part of the theatre, I didn't realize this, but I had dozed off during the last 15 minutes of his presentation. I woke up when the lights came on, looked around to some relief, thinking "good, no one noticed" my little unscheduled nap.

In his typical fashion, Dr. Lekic stood at the exit of the theatre, greeting each student as they left, thanking them for coming to his first lecture. Well, when I got to the door myself, he pulled me aside and in the gentlest manner saying the following to me (of course I'm paraphrasing, but I remember this like it was yesterday):

Him: "I felt so bad for you sitting there in the back."

Me: "Why is that, Dr. Lekic?" (Still a part of me hoping that he hadn't noticed me sleeping.)

Him: "Well, you didn't have a blanket. I know you've had a long week, and I don't blame you for that short nap, but I almost feel that if you're in my lecture I should care for you. I should have brought you a blanket and a pillow."

He didn't say it in a derogatory way or to embarrass me; he was being very genuine. And more so he said this to me privately. Now I've had the unfortunate luck of dozing off in other lectures in my years of university, and I've never been treated with this kindness. Most of the other professors made a habit of scolding me publicly in front of the other students. Shaming me. I even had a professor once kick me out of his theatre in front of over 150 people. But this man took a different approach, a kinder one, and 20 years later I still remember it like it was yesterday.

You can believe that I never fell asleep in his lectures ever again. That approach of *student-first* is what makes a professor the one you remember decades later, not the egotistic professors with the *how-dare-you-sleep-in-my-room* approach. And in my case specifically, he changed my life forever; I decided to follow in his footsteps.

—Fadi Kass, Class of 2002

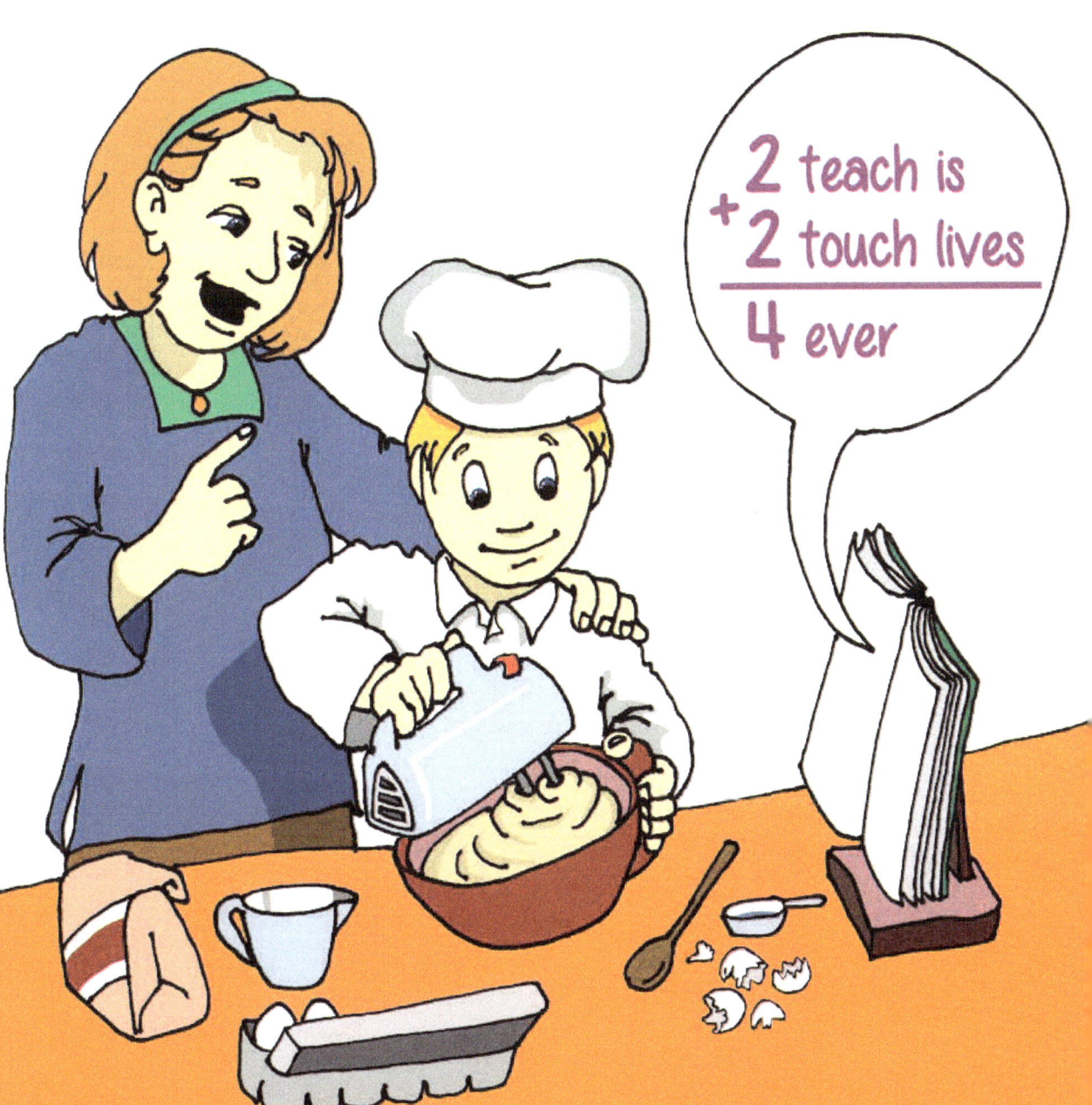

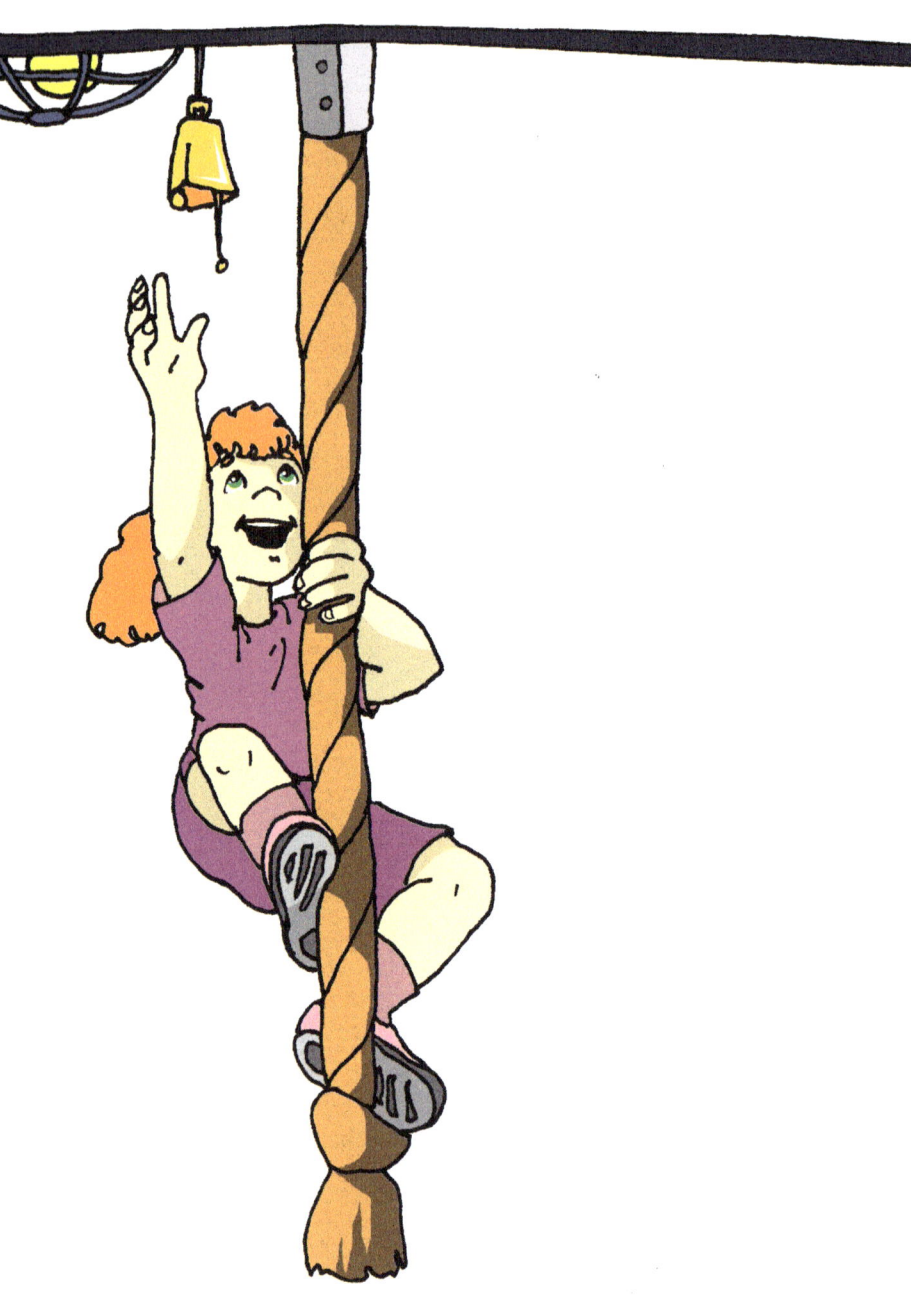

Optimism is the faith that leads to achievement.
Nothing can be done without hope and confidence.
—Helen Keller

Thank you for planting a seed.

Thank you for taking a seed of knowledge and planting it in the mind of a new student.

Thank you for watering that seed with warmth, explanation, demonstration, and inspiration.

Thank you for shining your care, concerns, encouragement, and optimism for the tiny seedling.

Thank you for nurturing, pruning, and tending to the curiosity and learning of the new tree.

Thank you for celebrating the flowers and fruit of the new tree as it began to express itself to those around.

Thank you for allowing this tree to make a difference in its world as you stand and smile in its shade.

Thank you for instilling in this tree the value of planting seeds of my own, caring for others, and seeing worth in others.

With much Appreciation and gratitude,
—Julie Maniate

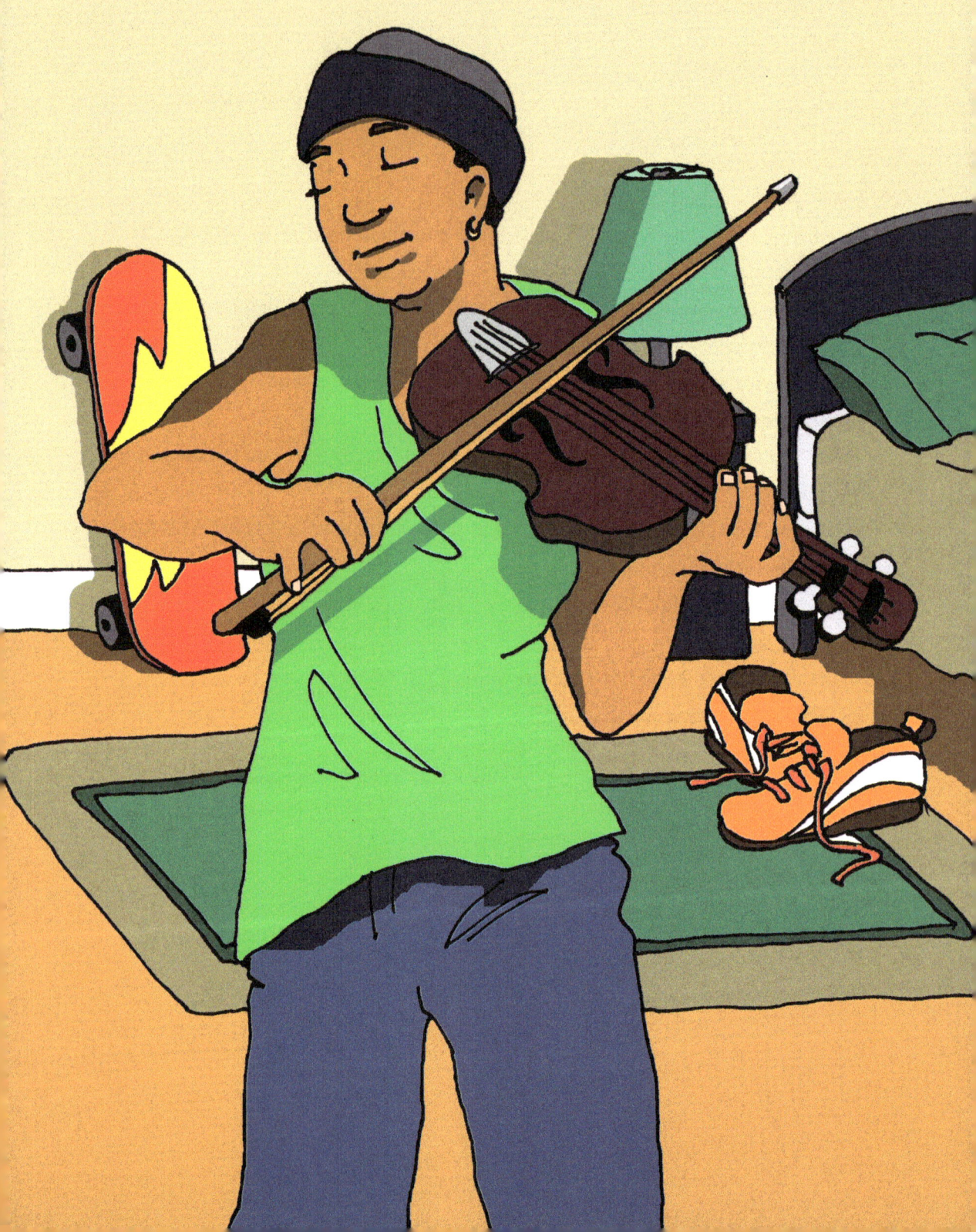

Quality means doing it right even when nobody is looking.
—Henry Ford

I first met Charles as he became our class advisor. Previous classes told us to think hard and to carefully choose our advisor, as that person would often have to stand up for the rights of our class. Charles showed all the qualities we thought that would represent us the best. We had no idea of what we were in for. He did much more than represent our class. He took time to help many with personal problems. He took the time to mentor us both within dentistry and life philosophy, most famously his beliefs in the power of caring. Within his role as advisor, he took on the rest of the university faculty in many situations where he thought there was an injustice. Many times at personal cost. When asked why he would take on personal adversities within the faculty to uphold what we thought was sometimes a more minor inconvenience, he would simply state, "because it is the right thing to do." That is what would most accurately sum him up, his deep integrity. Charles was more than an advisor to our class. He was our champion. Many professors take pride in their work, but Charles went beyond that and showed pride in people and much love, for which I will always be grateful.

—Robert Pesun

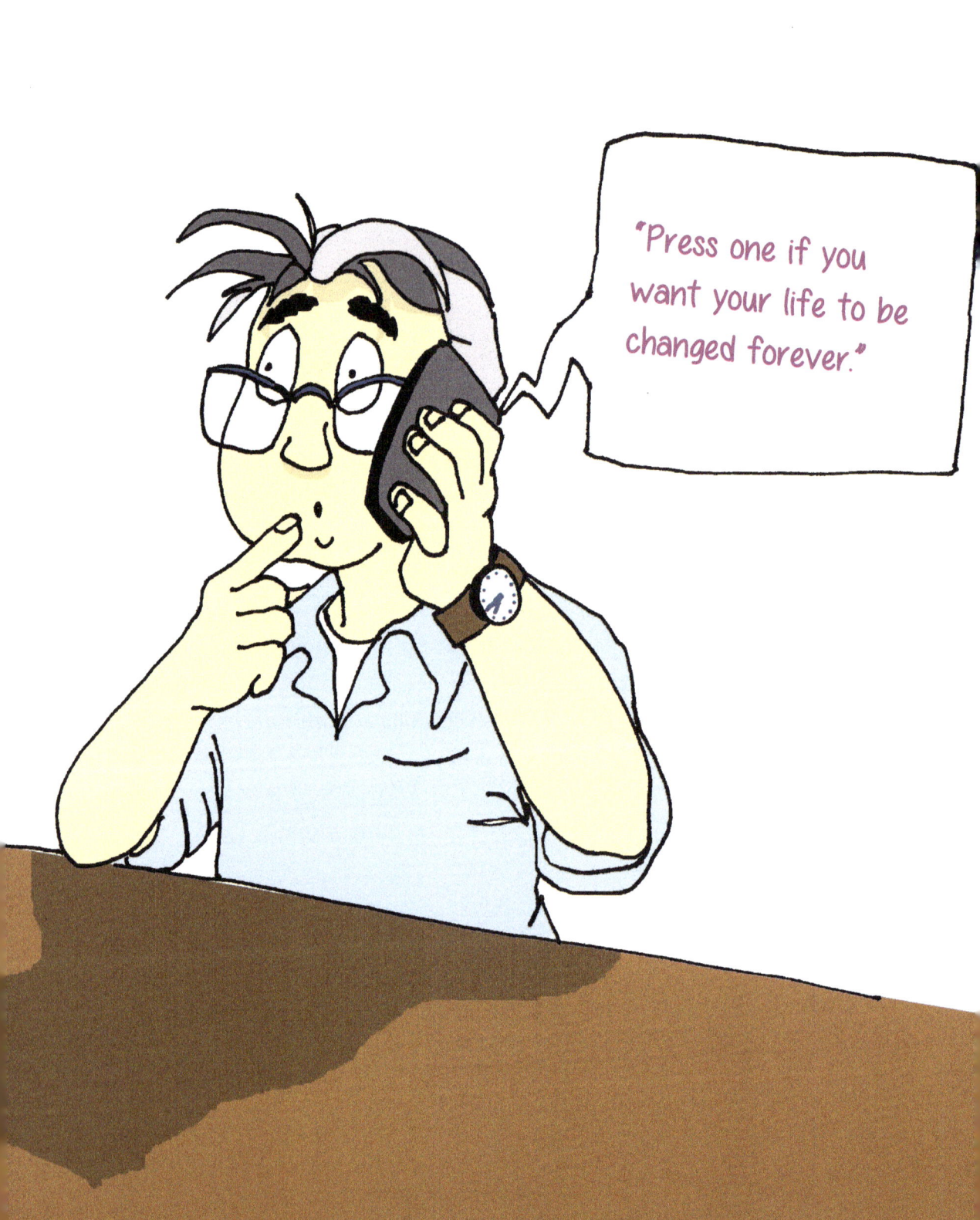

The phone call that changed a life.

Several years ago, I managed to find my way onto the website of the University of Manitoba College of Dentistry and saw that a new graduate program in Pediatric Dentistry was starting. I distinctly recall reading the description of the program and knew immediately that this was what I wanted to do. I immediately began organizing an application.

As luck would have it, I was granted an interview for admission into the program. I packed my dress clothes and began the long trek to Winnipeg. During the two-day process, I thought that I did everything that I could to put my best foot forward; the interviews seemed to go well, and I had no regrets. The program seemed like it would be awesome. Charles Lekic seemed like a person that I wanted to learn from.

Several weeks later came the bad news. Rejection. Didn't see that coming. Time to soul search. Time to move on?

I did move on. Life went on. The sun rose the next morning. I thought that it just "wasn't meant to be."

Then one day the following summer I got the phone call that changed my life. It was Charles Lekic on phone. We had a great conversation. Charles told me exactly why I wasn't successful and what I needed to do to improve. I was taken aback by the fact that he took the time to do this. He didn't have to do this. He gave me hope.

Where would I be if Charles would not have picked up the phone on that sunny day in July? Well, I can almost certainly say that I would not be a pediatric dentist. What a mistake that would have been to quit.

I was successful on my next application, and the rest is history. I have found a career that I love and am passionate about. What could be better than that?

I often wonder what life would be like if Charles did not call me that day, but then I quickly realize that he did call that day and that is all that matters. That 10-minute phone call truly did change a life. For that I am eternally grateful."

—Mark Berscheid

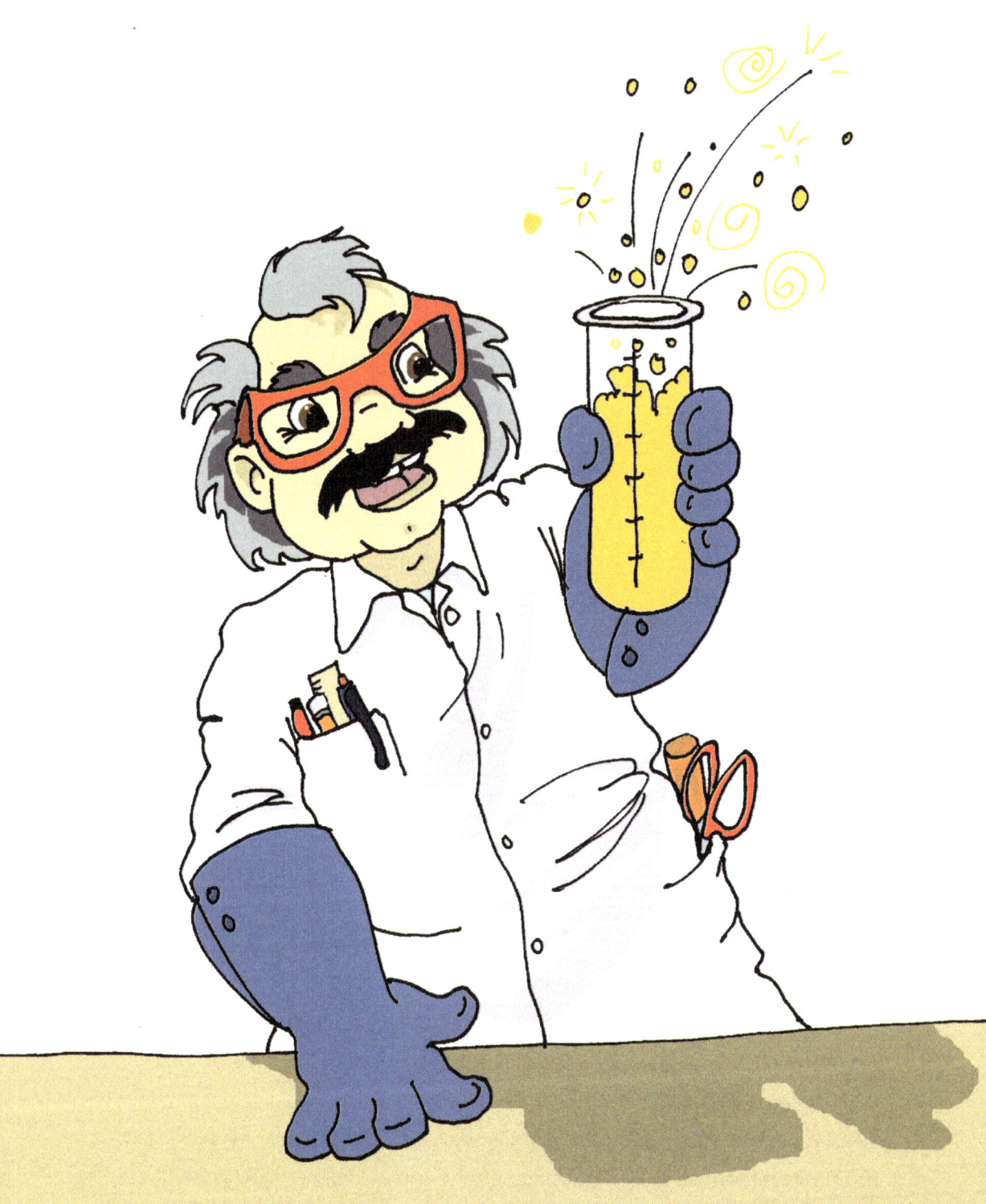

I'm not crazy because I teach.
I'm just crazy about being a teacher!

Teaching

Hi Dr. Lekic,

I just wanted to extend a big thank you for choosing to celebrate your retirement with all of your students and friends/family. The Fort Garry put on a wonderful dinner and thanks for inviting us.

I also just wanted to say thank you for always having our backs during our four years in dental school. You were extremely kind and generous to our class over the four years that you acted as our class advisor. You invited us into your home and fed us and gave us wine; it was always a lovely treat.

We truly could see that no matter what, you put the students first. You supported our ideas and always stood beside us when we put up a stand towards faculty issues.

Thanks for treating us like family. I wish you well in the years to come and hope you can find some time to relax!

Sincerely,

—Darci Bonar, Class of 2011

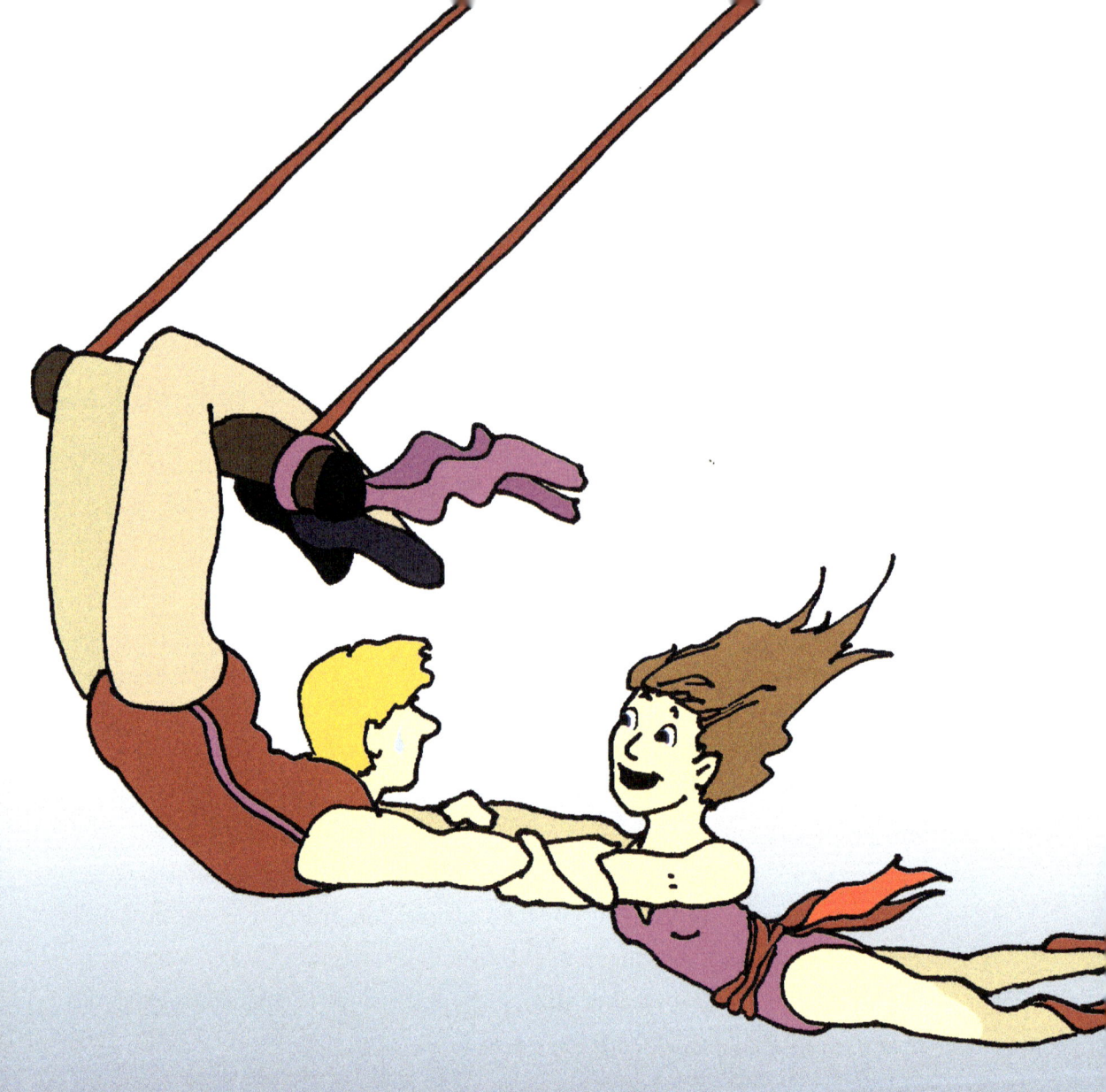

We rise by lifting others.

A true teacher is someone who teaches his pupils beyond the confines of a classroom. He influences his students to be better members of society. He teaches the importance of giving back to others and how this is the true meaning of success. When one has a teacher with these qualities, these values resonate throughout their lifetime and make the world a better place. Thank you, Dr. Charles Lekic, for being my teacher.

—Omar Mohammad,
Class of 2009

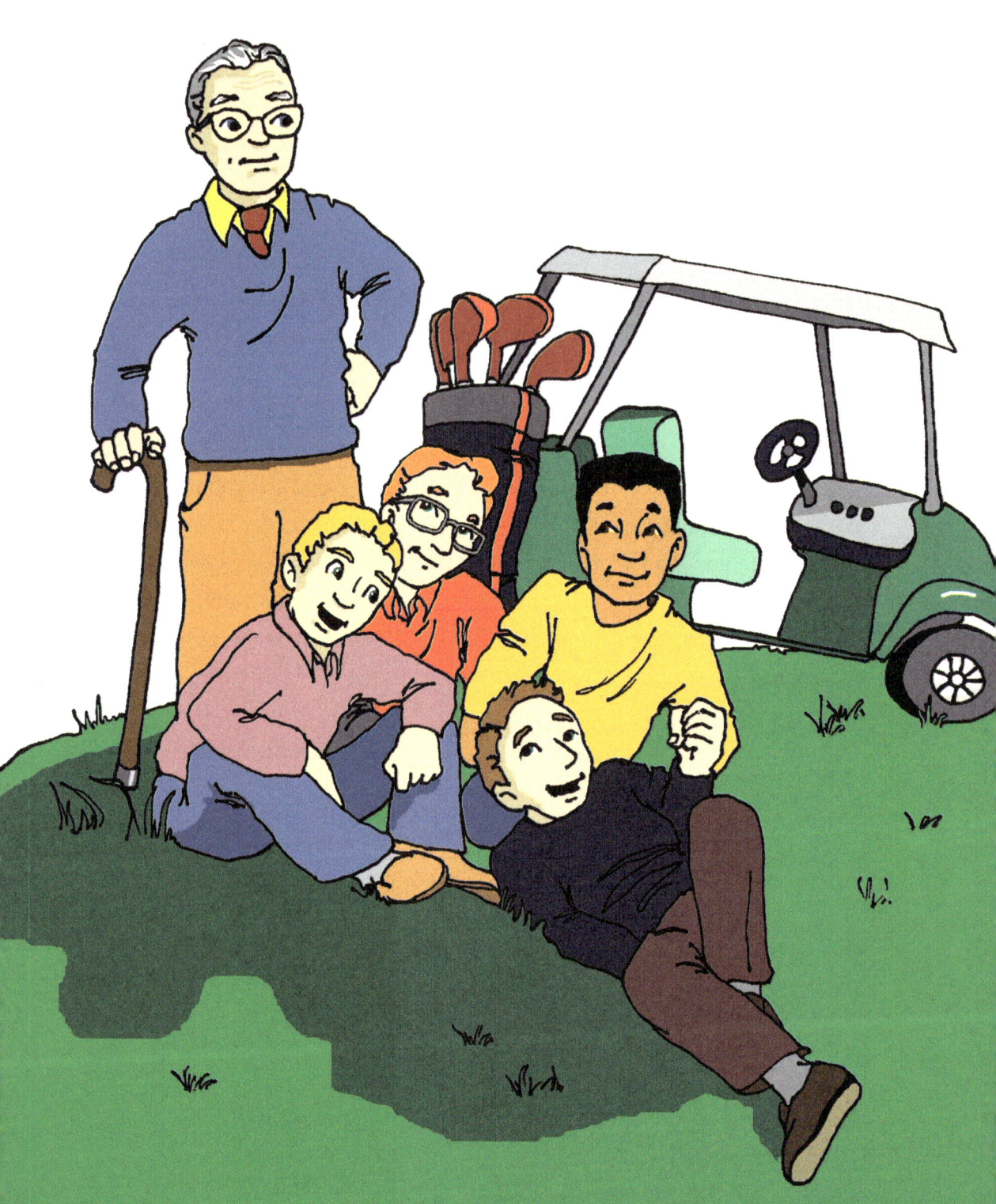

Even 10 days after surgery,
it's expected for the instructor to be with the students.

My personal experience in dental school was a very positive one. I often look back at those four years as one of the best periods of my life. A lot of learning, a lot of hard work, but also a lot of friendships and good memories. Yes, there were tough times and some instructors that weren't positive, but a lot of good, positive, caring, supportive instructors as well. Dr Charles Lekic was definitely one of the most positive instructors I've ever had. When the instructor is positive, supportive, and generally happy to be teaching, it shows. Not only that, but it also motivates the student to do better and work harder. All that in an environment that has no negative pressure and tension. Dr Lekic also made himself available to students outside of the school, time which is important. To get to know your instructor outside of the school element is not only nice, but also is needed to nurture the bond and accountability between instructors and students. I truly believe that there is more than just teaching to be a good teacher. You have to genuinely care about your work and about your students, and Dr Lekic did just that.

—Alex Serebnitski

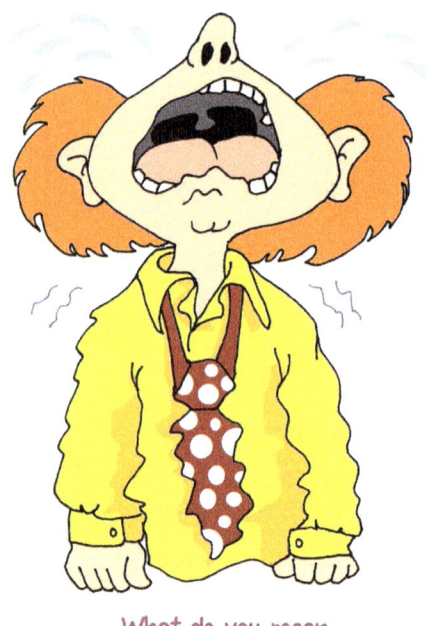

What do you mean I have to be good? Don't I get weekends off?

Dear Charles,

It was such an honour to celebrate with you and so many others your retirement from the university. Twenty years well spent. Where does the time go? Time that has seen me transition from your student to your colleague and more importantly from a stranger to your friend. Throughout these changes, I have always admired your pursuit of excellence and the many areas you have achieved it in – enthusiasm and tremendous teacher, clinician, researcher. Roles you have embraced with energy! In doing so, you have done much to encourage and inspire me in my own career, as I know you have done for countless others. Thank you. So even as your time at the university ends, I know that your desire to invest in others professional and personally, will not. Looking back, your successes have been many; may they continue and multiply as you enter this next season of post-academic life.

—From your student turned friend,

Jay Biber

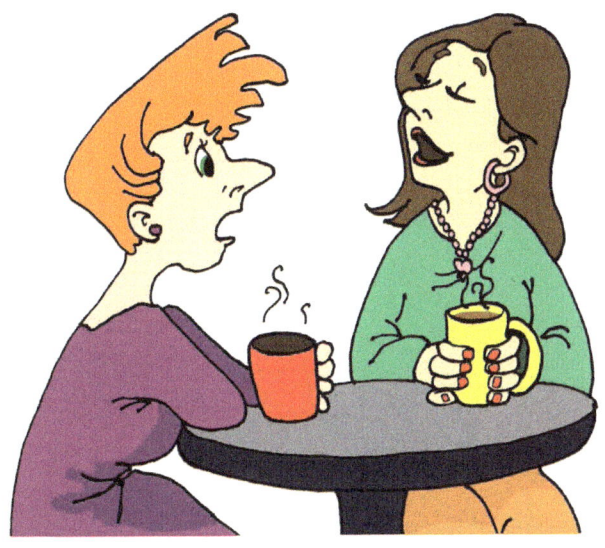

"You get along with everyone, what's your secret?"

"Nobody hates a listener!"

Three things that I hold dear to me which I have learned from Dr. Lekic, which I use in private practice and life in general:

1. Always be a good listener. Listen to the questions and concerns of the patient and parents and answer them before starting any procedure.

2. Never lie to a patient, especially a child. Don't tell him/her that a procedure is "not going to hurt at all." Their trust in you will be broken, which is very difficult or even impossible to rebuild.

3. You can always find flaws in people, but you should always look at the good first.

—Harpreet Sroay

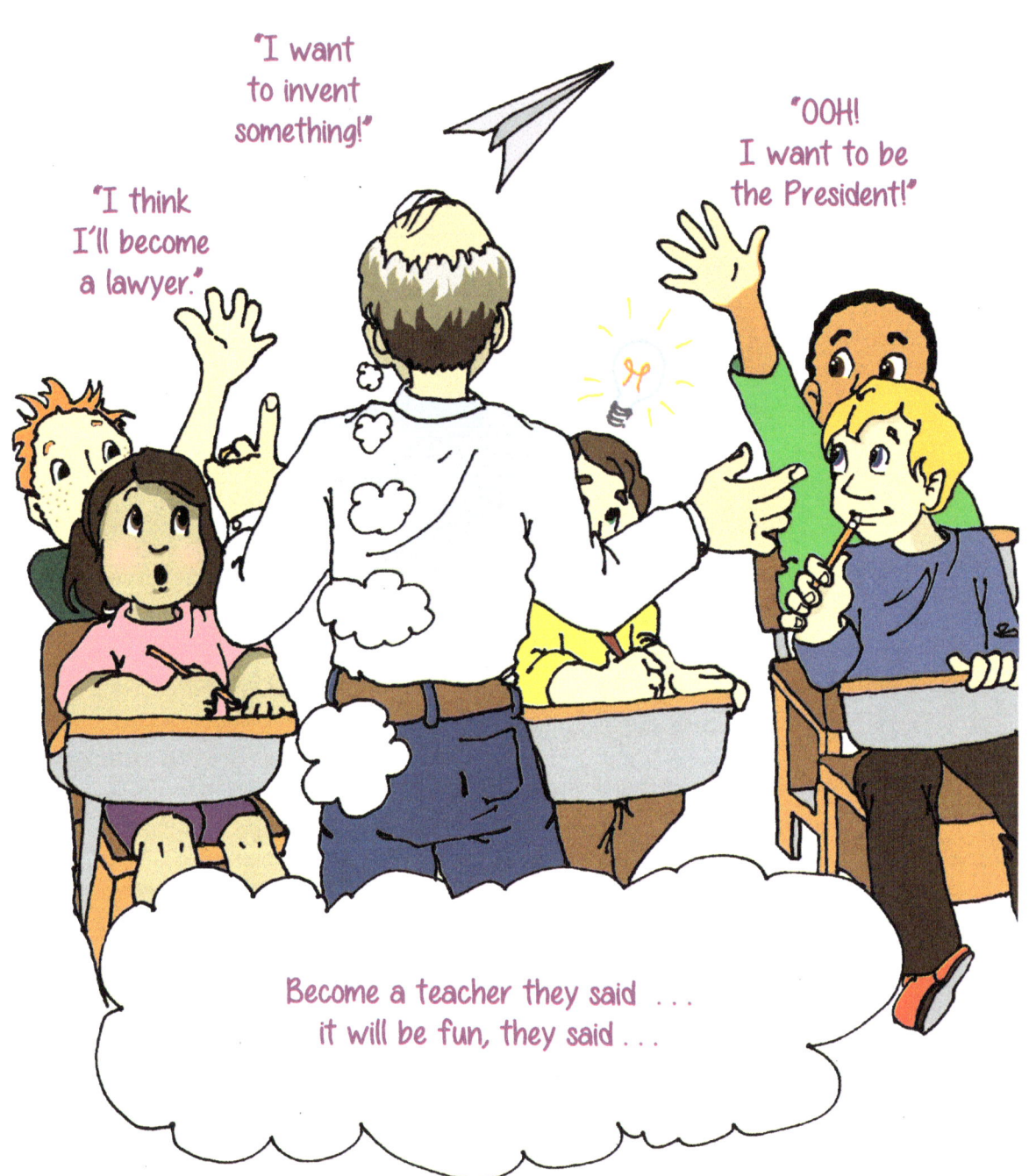

Teaching is the ultimate form of giving.

The first time I met Charles, I was an applicant to the graduate pediatric dentistry program in Manitoba. He made a lasting impression on me because he was humble and insisted on us calling him by his first name only. He spoke about the importance of giving back to the community, and because I have a background in working with under-privileged people, these ideals resonated with me. After an evening out with his residents and hearing them speak about their program and its director, I knew that the Manitoba program was right for me.

It is rare to find an individual who has committed their life's work to academia, while at the same time maintaining a successful practice. Watching Charles balance these two things has been inspirational and has shown me that he truly does believe in giving back to his community. Dedicating so much time in your career to academia is truly the ultimate form of giving back. Being an educator is a gift to the community because, moved by the teacher, many of the dentists will go out into their own communities with the same ideals and will help an even broader population. Some will even be inspired to commit more time to teaching as well.

When Charles announced he was retiring, I remember looking around the room and, based on all the teary eyes that I saw, I knew what a huge loss to our program it would be. Despite being around less, Charles has promised his residents that he will continue to make himself available to us, which was immensely reassuring to us all.

I wish you the very best in your retirement, Charles.

—Jennifer Coutu

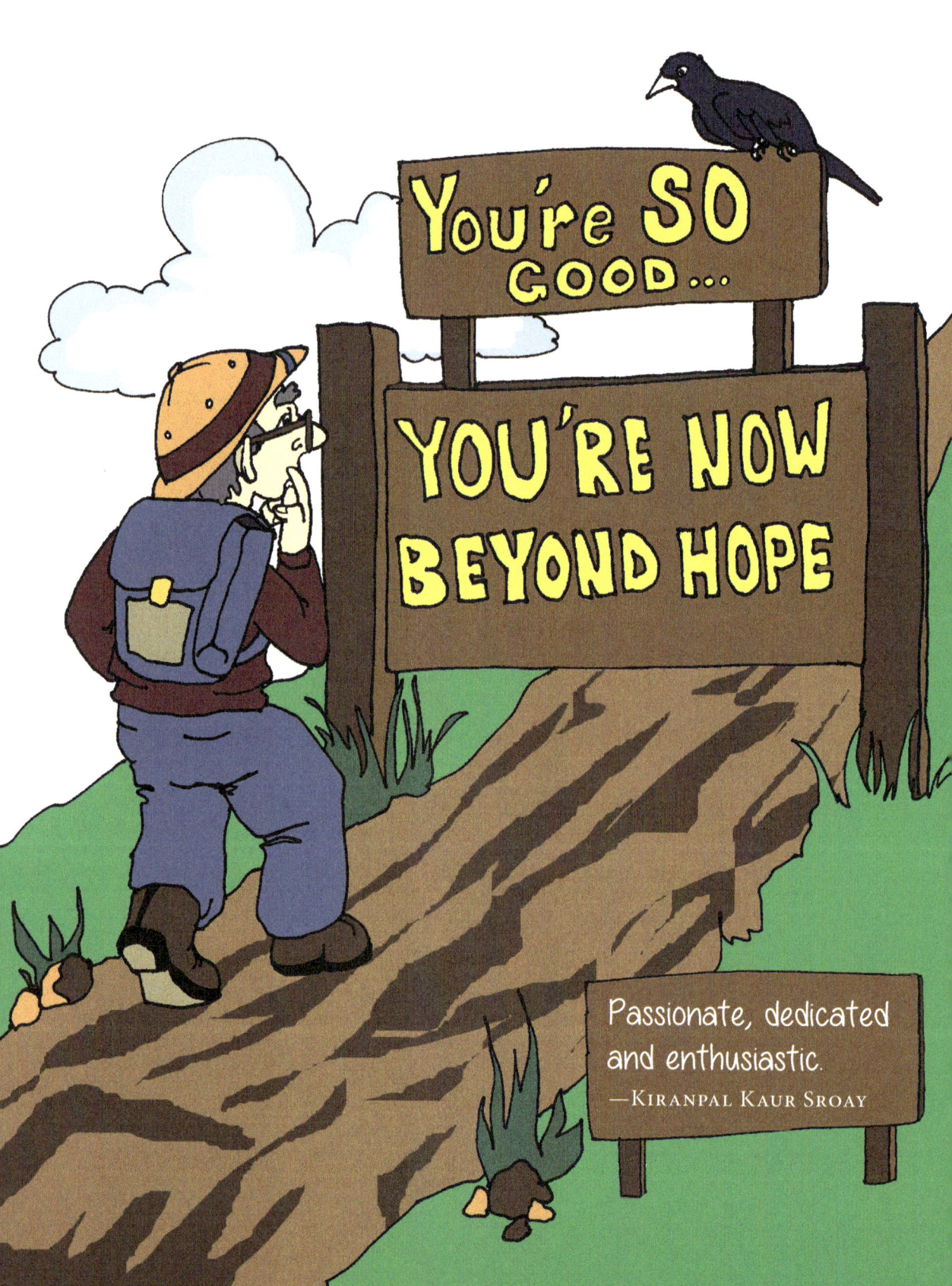

Passionate, dedicated and enthusiastic.
—Kiranpal Kaur Sroay

My experiences with Dr. Charles Lekic as both his student and now as his colleague over the past 12 years I've known him have been incredible. These experiences have shaped my future by inspiring me to become a pediatric dentist and taught me the importance of caring for others, especially patients and colleagues, as dear members of my own family.

I first met Charles when I was an undergraduate dental student at the University of Manitoba and he was the head of the undergraduate pediatric dentistry program. I and my classmates all looked forward to Fridays, not just because they were the end of a hard school week, but because Fridays were pedo clinic, and we knew we would be working with Charles. His enthusiasm for treating children and his commitment to teaching us to also love providing dental care for children is the sole reason I decided to become a pediatric dentist. It is safe to say his caring spirit inspired me, and his silly jokes brought some lightness and fun to my schooling. He taught my dental class to do our absolute best for every single patient and treat every child as if they were part of our family. He also encouraged a silly and fun side to interacting with children, such as singing to them or telling funny stories. Charles always has a funny story to tell in any scenario, and he is also the first person to make fun of himself, often bringing those around him to uncontrollable laughter. It was through these positive experiences in undergraduate pedo clinic that I decided to become a pediatric dentist, since I wanted to make a difference in children's lives in the way I saw Charles and his team of pediatric dentistry professors do.

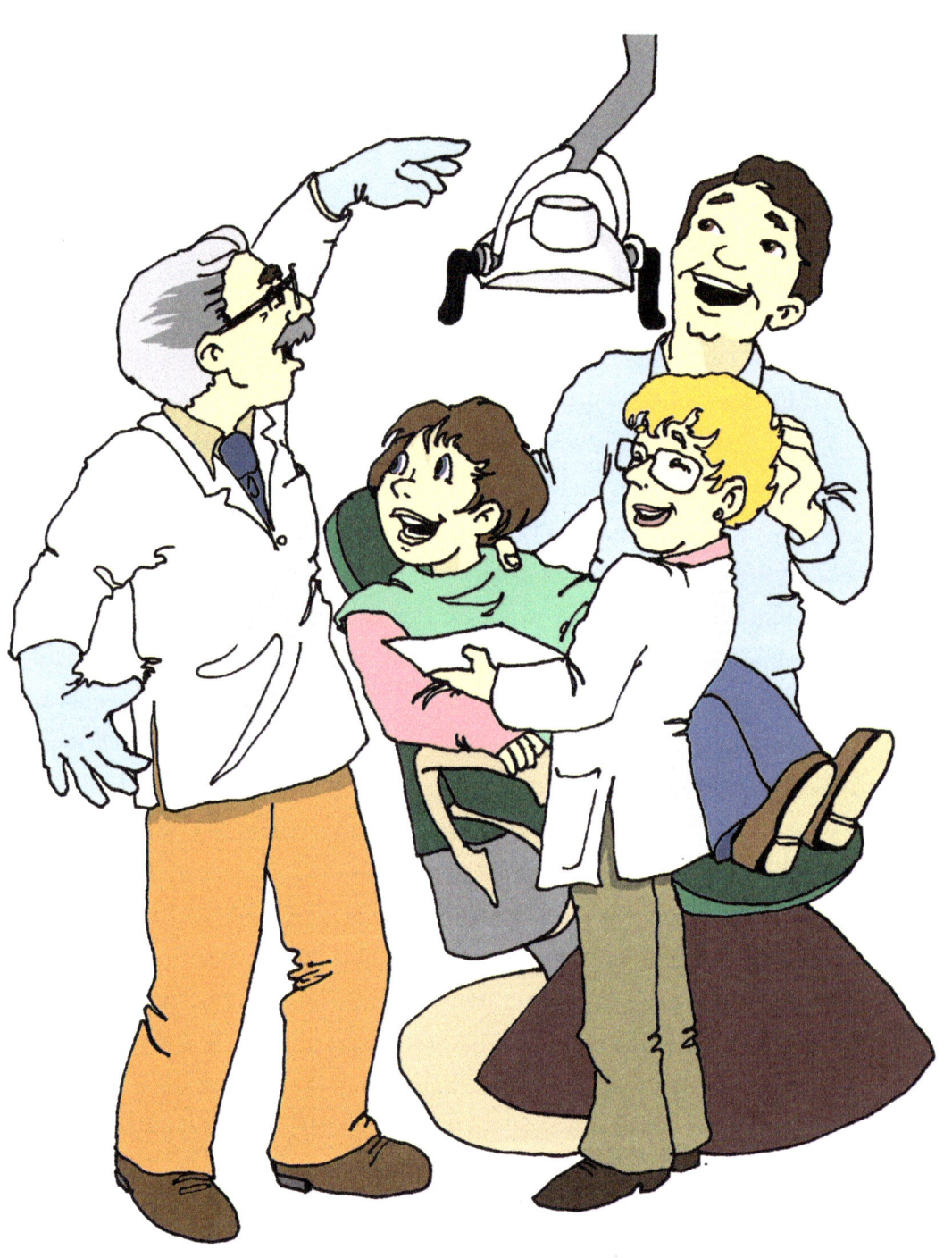

How to tell a funny story.

Charles went on to achieve the great accomplishment of opening a graduate pediatric dentistry Masters program at the University of Manitoba, doing the majority of writing and preparation for the program while he was recovering from back surgery. I think this is a testament to the fact that, if you believe in something and commit all your effort to it, anything is possible. This is another lesson Charles has taught me. As a resident in the program starting in the second year it existed, I saw Charles generously donate enormous amounts of his personal time to get the program started and ensure its survival and also large amounts of his personal funds. He was always available to residents for questions or seminars on evenings or weekends, and he was never too busy for his students. I can remember being a first year resident on call for the hospital and calling Charles very late at night with a question about a trauma that had arrived at the emergency room. He answered his phone right away and did not make me feel bad for waking him up so late at night (which may have been the reaction for most people receiving a late-night phone call from their student), but instead he gave me advice and asked if I'd like him to meet me at the emergency room to help with the trauma case. This is one example of how Charles always made his residents feel like we could ask him anything at any time, and he would always give us his full attention.

I have many silly stories too from my time as a resident with Charles as my program director. He wanted to teach the residents the importance of being on time for our commitments (another important life lesson I learned from Charles), and so he started a fund that if a resident was late to clinic or a meeting, they would put $25 into, and it would be used every so often to buy all the residents coffee or pizza (or whatever the residents decided to use the money for). However, Charles, being the amazing teacher he is, also made the rule that if he was late, he would pay $50 to the same fund. I think this was to teach us that no matter who you are, resident or program director, you should always value others' time. Needless to say, we have some funny stories of Charles being late, the most commonly recurring theme being that he spilt his coffee (again)! I think Charles was the only contributor to this "late fund," and he paid his dues every time with a smile.

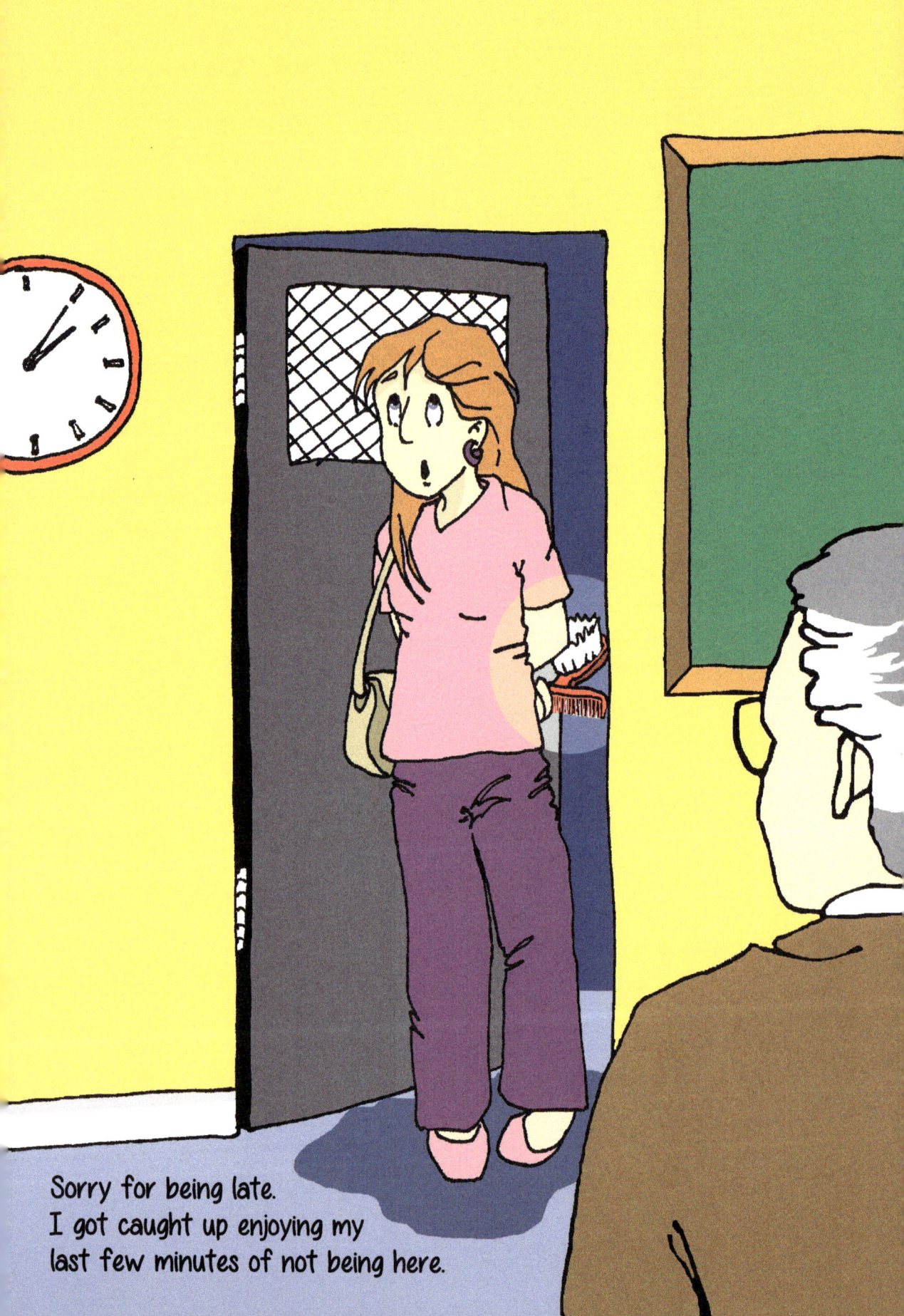

I now work with Charles in private practice and have seen first-hand his dedication to his patients and also to growing the practice. As a new graduate, he has acted as my mentor, and even though he has officially retired from the university, I still consider him my teacher since I often ask him for advice, and I still learn so much from him. I think Charles will continue to teach and mentor others his whole life because that's part of who he is: a caring individual who genuinely wants to make the world a better place and wants to help everyone in his life be the best person they can be. I feel so blessed to have had such an extraordinary teacher in my life who has inspired me to become the person I am today, and I am happy to say that I consider Charles a friend for life. Thank you, Charles, for all you have done for your students and the University of Manitoba. I know many lives have been touched by your hard work and that you've done so much good for our university and the next generation of dental professionals.

—Amanda Huminicki

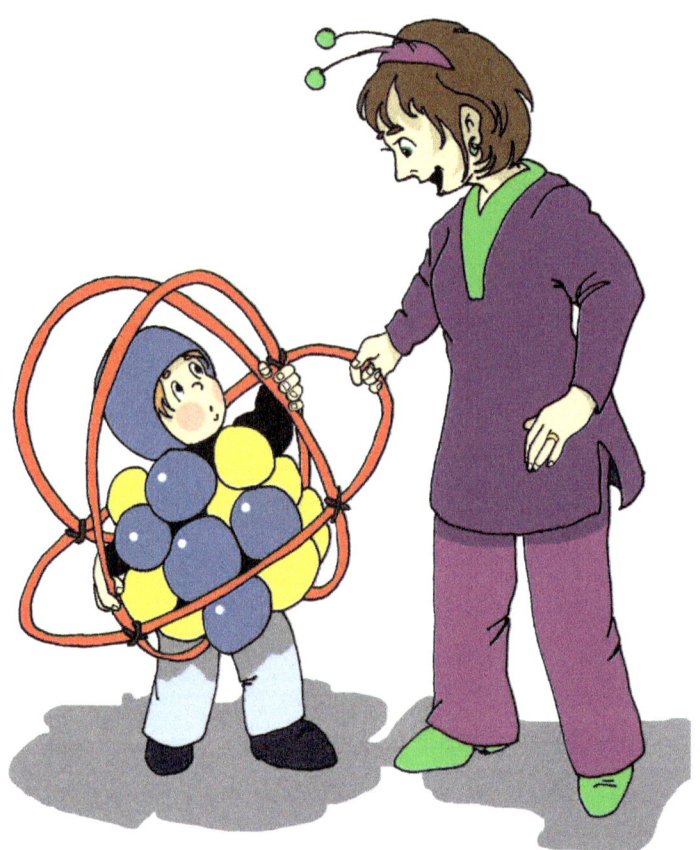

Think like a proton and stay positive!

"Deeper Teaching promotes Deeper Learning"

At the time of writing these thoughts, I have known Dr. Charles Lekic for only a short period — a little over a year. But it became obvious from our initial interaction as a student/teacher that he embraces the utmost important educational philosophy of "Deeper Teaching promotes Deeper Learning".

Deeper teaching involves fully engaging the student as an equal partner in the experience of learning. From the first time I was included in an educational discussion with Charles, it involved much less "teacher talk" and more educational discussion – educational discussion containing equal amounts of clinical experience and scientific research.

"Deeper Learning" should be the goal of all students, but it can only be achieved through the process of "Deeper Teaching" and by one who is willing to push the boundaries of conventional instruction, encouraging the student to be actively involved in the educational process, an equal partner without fear of failure or embarrassment due to lack of knowledge. Deeper teaching in dentistry (as in all patient-based health fields) involves both clinical practicality and supportive scientific research with the ultimate goal to further dentistry as a "clinical, research-based profession".

In the relatively short time period I have known Charles, I have come to appreciate the concept of "Deeper Teaching promotes Deeper Learning" as something he excels at and is a model for future educators and mentors. I have come to appreciate the importance of scientific-based research education and its importance to our profession. Without supportive scientific research, our profession of dentistry would not be able to flourish.

Practice must not rest upon experiment but upon science, a professional education is presumably a scientific education. The trades are learned by practical methods alone, but the professions are acquired by the study of the sciences involved. We (Dentistry) claim to be a profession; therefore, let our education be scientific that we may justify the claim. Let us guard the scientific branches as the vital part of our education, to lose which would be to lose all.

—Excerpt from the speech "Scientific Instruction in Our Colleges"
by A.H. Thompson D.D.S. Chicago, IL

Dr. Charles Lekic exemplifies the importance of sound, scientific, research-based education and the importance of safeguarding our profession through the furthering of science-based clinical education and research. It is through his thoughtful "Deeper Teaching" that I am able to enjoy a "Deeper Learning" of our profession.

—CAMERON GRANT
Pediatric Dental Resident / University of Manitoba
July 25, 2016

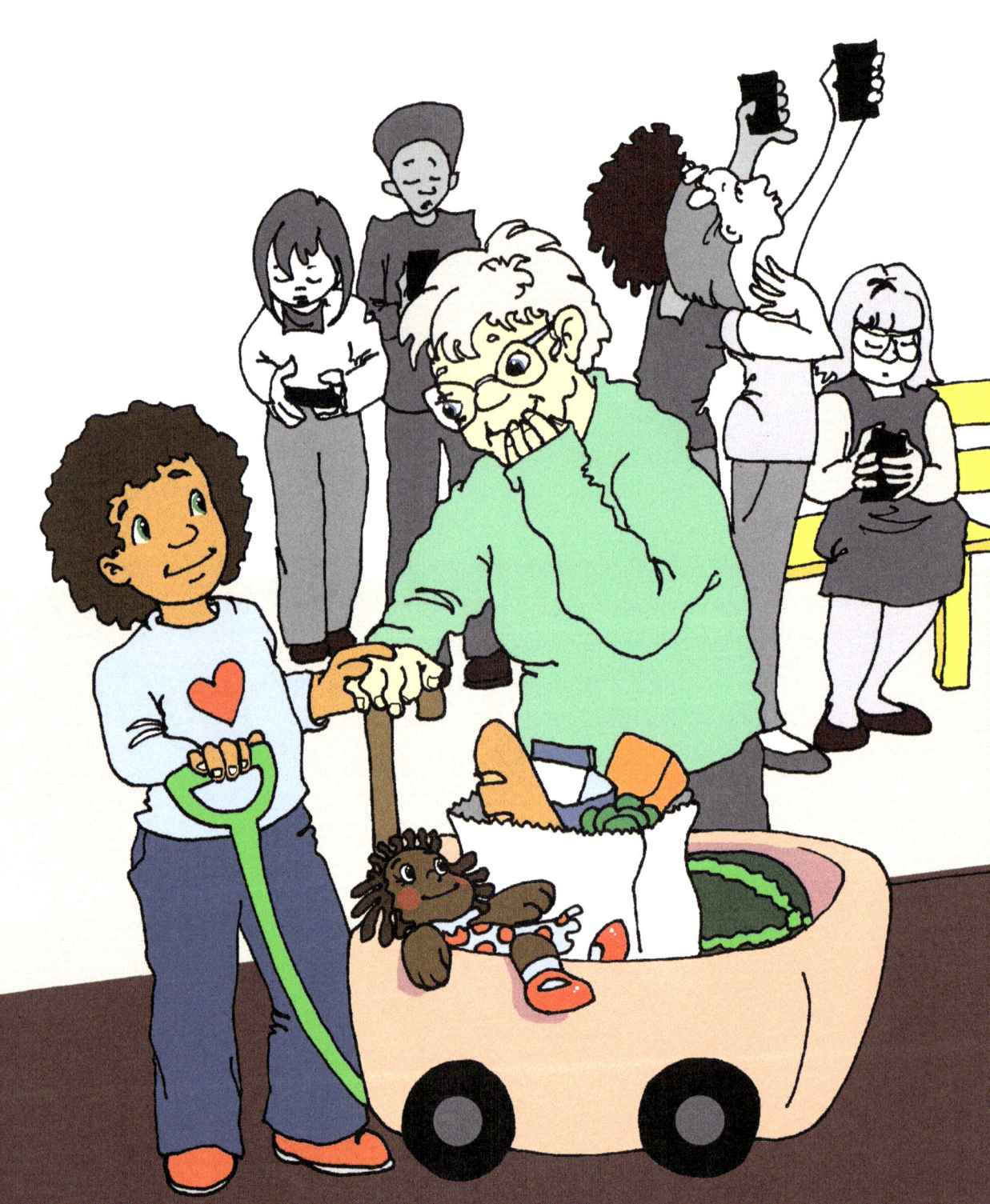

If you desire to make a difference in the world, you must be different!

A Journey

I would say my experience as a pediatric dental resident in Charles' program has been a journey – one that I am still currently on.

It started on the day of my interview at the U of M. I was just amazed by the program director that had given his welcome speech. He was so humble and down to earth. He mentioned how important it was to give back to the community and to work with your heart and not your head. He explained these were the core values for his program and how here in Manitoba the program is a family. This was the family I wanted to be a part of. I had just interviewed at another school, which was at the time my frontrunner. But after day one of my U of M interview experience, that had all changed, and I wanted to come to the U of M for pediatric dentistry.

Luck would have it that I got both offers and chose to continue my journey at the U of M. I would say I was disappointed when Charles left for his sabbatical – but let's be honest, it was not easy for him to stay away. After all, the program was his child, and he always nurtured it well. I saw firsthand Charles being the students' advocate that he is well known for. He fought hard for the program to be recognized and accepted into PARIMs so that his residents would be treated as equals amongst the medical residents. He is a true warrior.

Charles was my advisor on my thesis committee. He had his 'golden rule' that no matter how busy he was, which city he was in, he would always read and edit my rough copies within 24 hours. This was his guarantee, and he always managed to do it.

Charles has *always* had an open-door policy. He always listened to our concerns, and even if he didn't agree, he would listen and explain the reasoning behind his decision. I have always felt comfortable at my program, knowing that we had a program director willing to listen and make our experience here the best he could possibly make it.

I can say that the journey is still continuing even though he says he will retire. I know he will always be there for his residents, and I take great comfort in that.

Thank you, Charles, for being the most wonderful mentor for your residents.

—Anonymous

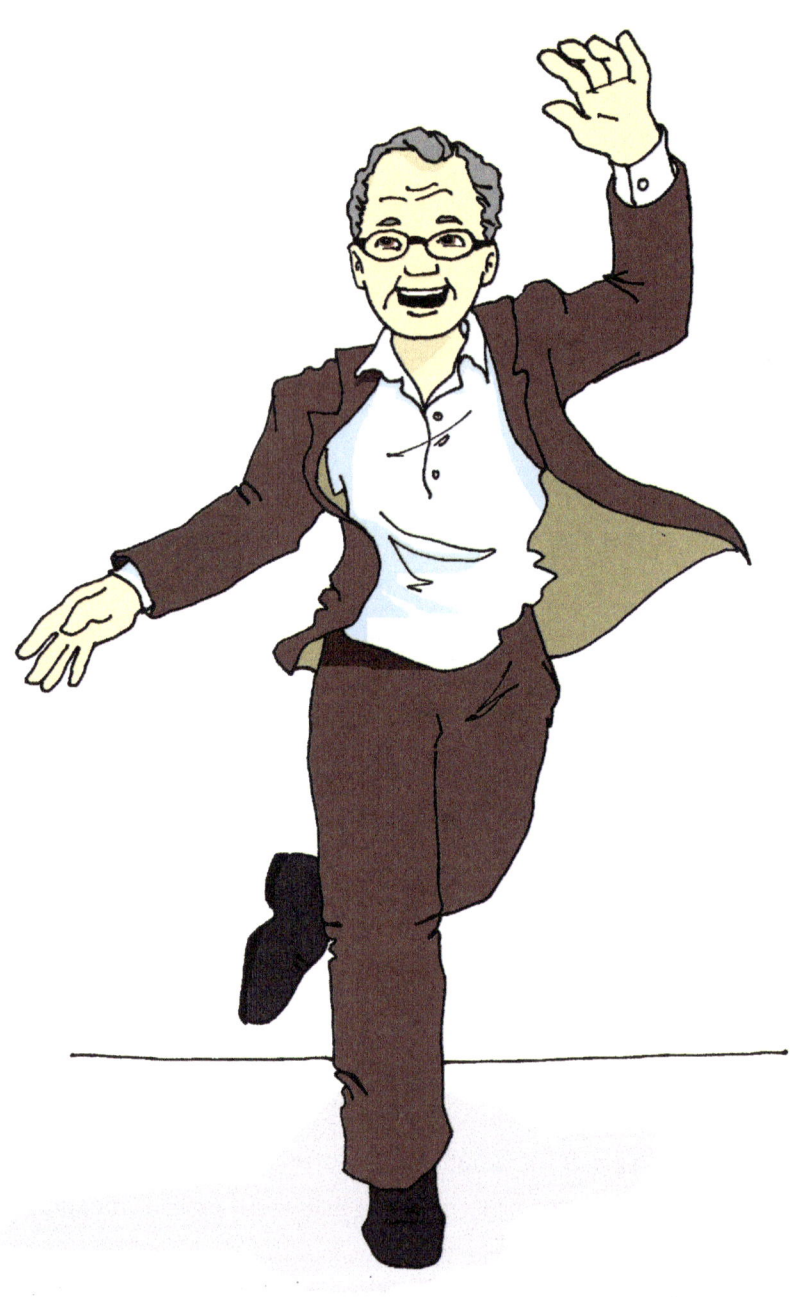

Always happy and smiley.

I met Charles' son Milos before I met him. The friendliest, smiley ball of stress. A type of guy you cannot help but love. He was in my dental class. As the weeks in the first year went on, I learned that his father is one of the professors at the school and that he would not be a part of the program for our class due to conflict of interest. We got a young female as the instructor. And it was great until I graduated dental school and came back to help out in the undergraduate pediatric clinic on Fridays. This is when I truly got to know Charles. He took me under his wing and restored my faith in the dental community and humanity in general! And it is then that I realized how much my class missed out ...

The first Friday I came back to the dental school, I was very nervous. It was as though I was writing a final exam. All the memories from the dental school came flooding in. Trust me, it was not pleasant! However, Charles was in the clinic with his usual smile waiting for us all. He was so passionate about his job, his colleagues, students, and the advancements in our field. I remember that first day he showed me the two rooms that were set up and designed specifically for children with autism. I had no idea what autism is, and I for sure was not going to ask him. You did not ask questions in the dental school I came from. His fervor made me secretly look up autism on the clinic computer, and I realized how much ahead of the game he is than anyone I know. By the end of the day, I came to know that Charles is not the typical professor we have had throughout the dental school, and that the biggest mistake I made that day was not the fact that I did not know what autism was, but that I did not ask him.

Close to the end of that school year, he came up to me and asked, "What are your plans for the future?" During dental school I wanted to specialize in Oral Surgery; however, last year in dental school made me realize this is not for me. We talked all afternoon. His words reminded me so much of my grandfather, whom I called "Deedoh", who passed away just a year before. My grandfather was a teacher and always caring, but most of all honest and to the point. He, just like Charles, always pushed people to do better. That afternoon Charles made his point for sure, and changed my life forever. Two and a half years later, I graduated as a pediatric dentist. To this day when I think of him, I think of my grandfather, and my heart just swells with love and affection.

—Edina Heder

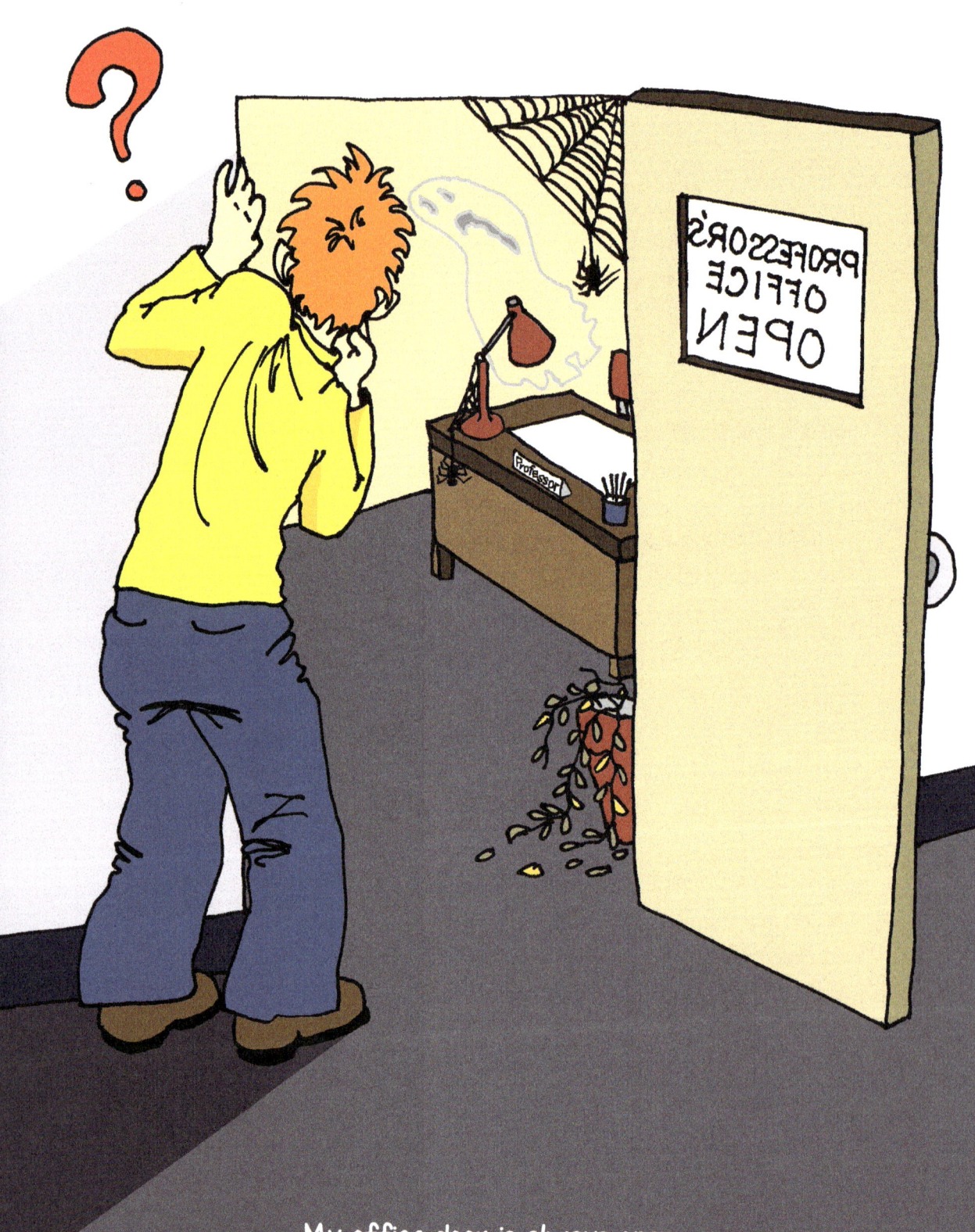

My office door is always open . . .
however, I'm rarely there.

Dr Lekic

An Engager. An Educator. An Inspirer. These three characteristics are just a short sample of the many you demonstrate with all of your students, including me, every single day.

Too often we progress through the 'ropes of life,' and do not invest the time to express our gratitude and appreciation for the support you so eagerly share for our growth, as not only students, but also to the dental community in large.

You make me feel truly supported when you say, "My door is always open, please just come in" and genuinely mean it. Also, the excitement you express to teach and mentor me makes me feel like a colleague in my learning experience. I know you have so much to share, but I love how you also openly articulate how much I have to share as well and how much you learn by engaging with me!

As an educator, your title can ensure a role of heightening my knowledge in academics. However, you see me not as one of the many students you have, but instead you treat me like family. You promote an environment where I feel like I am able to not only share my contribution, but also know it is actually considered and appreciated.

Thank you for being genuine and caring. Thank you for seeing me as a colleague in learning and sharing. Thank you for being you. Thank you for being one of the few great teachers out there. May you inspire others to achieve the greatness you have.

With gratitude,
SHERIF ELSARAJ, DENT 2010 CLASS PRESIDENT

Part Two
Staff

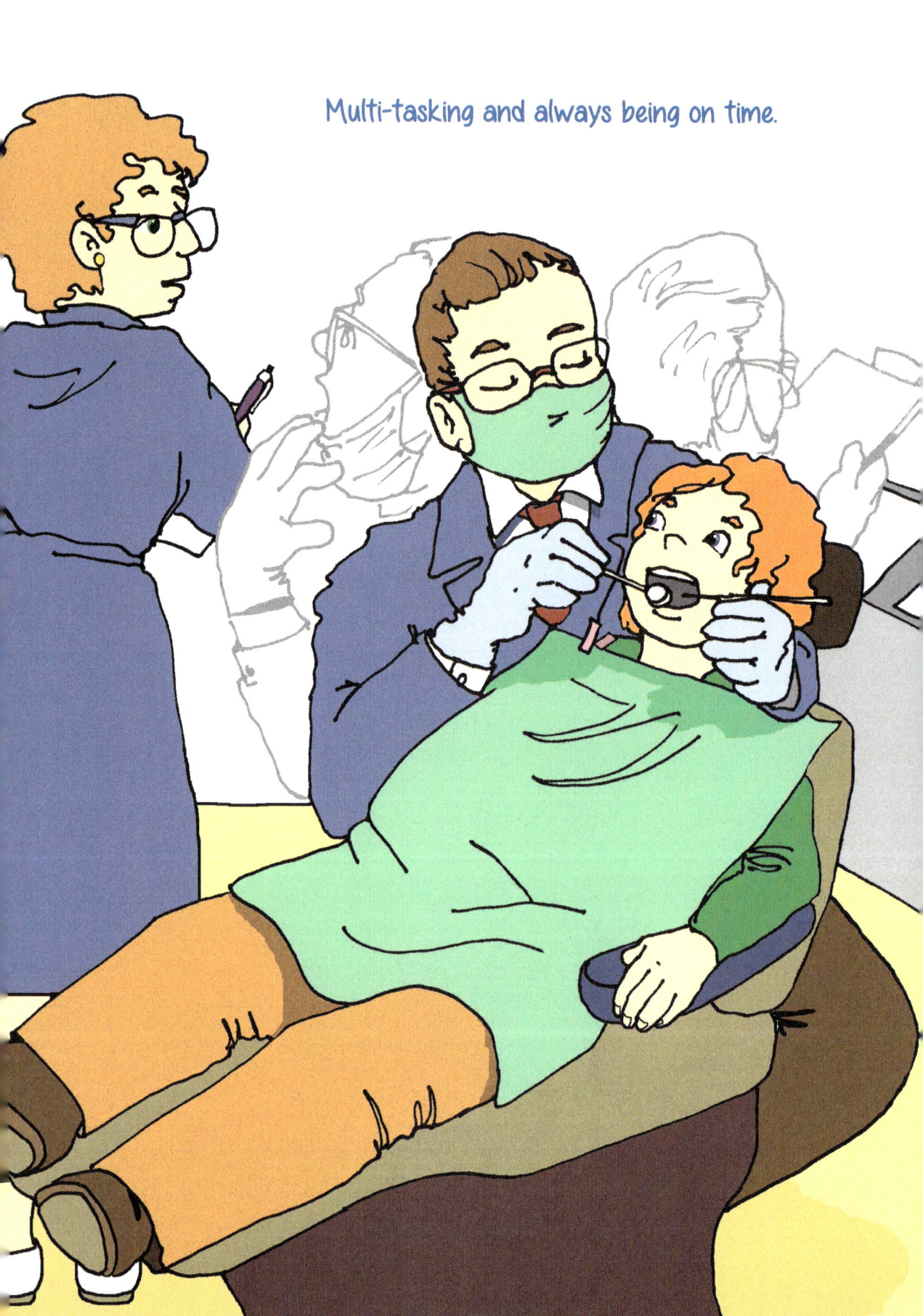
Multi-tasking and always being on time.

Working with less than 10 years

A true teacher. The only dentist I have worked with in 30 years that can actually work faster and more focused, the more he talks and explains. Thank you, Charles, for sharing your knowledge.

—Diane Mymko

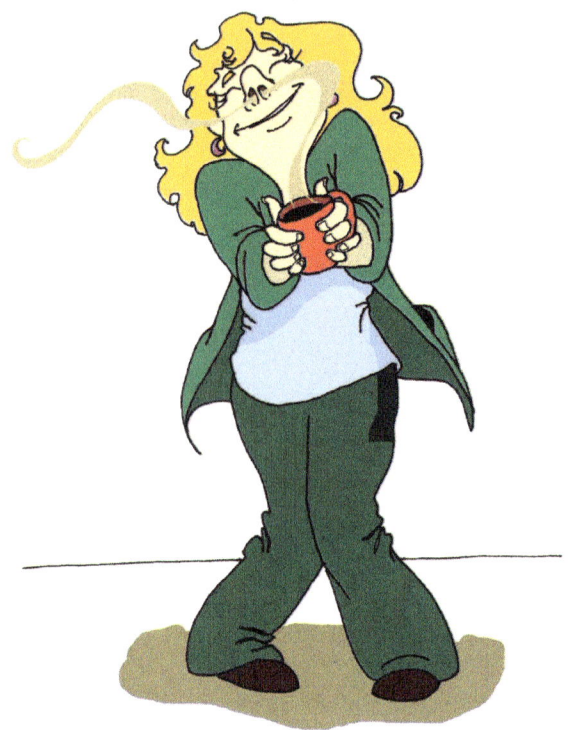

You had me at "coffee!"

The one thing that I noticed with Charles is that he really takes note of little details about a person. For example: in our office he learnt early on that we all appreciate a cup of coffee. He would go for coffee and have remembered how we all like to drink our beverage. That's what stands out for me the most. I want to add that the residents have noticed your absence; however, there is one thing I don't miss, and that is your singing. Maybe now you will have time to join Julie when she goes for her voice lessons. At the end one thing I would like to say is that you are very easy to talk to. Thanks for that.

—Val Friesen

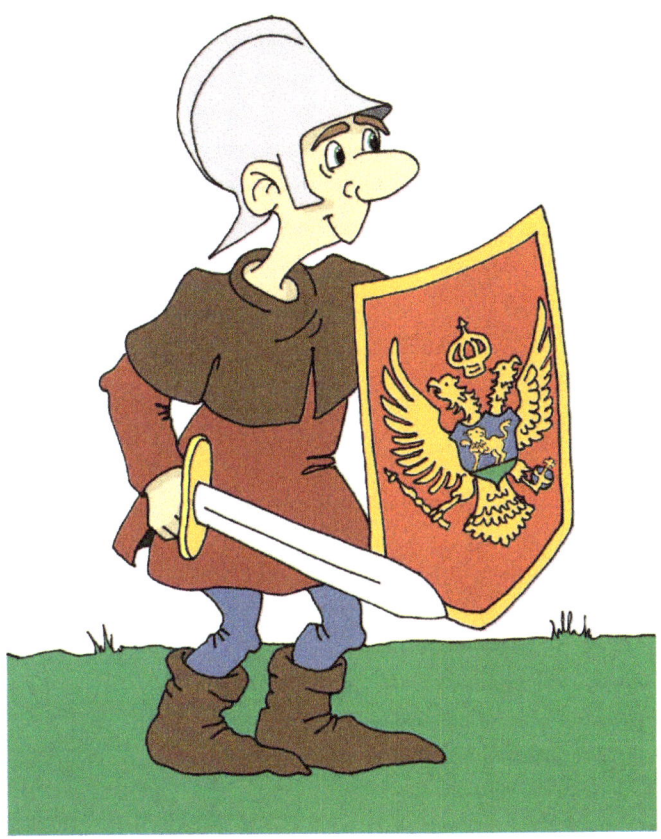

I remember the time I first joined the University of Manitoba. I was like a wide-eyed child in a big, unknown world. Charles was always there to guide me through this hard, life-transforming journey. Since the beginning we realized we had a lot in common, both immigrants, both passionate pediatric dentists. Together, we shared my failures and triumphs. His experience and support were my guidance and essential components of my professional life.

As one can imagine, having Charles as my boss was not always easy. He is the type of person that wants always the best possible outcome of everything: do it right or don't do it. Those who know him well know he is a genius, and his personality made me a better professional. I have no words to describe how important he is to myself, my family, and my career. Charles is a warrior who fights with his life for his beliefs and beloveds. I am so thankful for having had the opportunity to work with him and be his friend.

—Adriana Salles

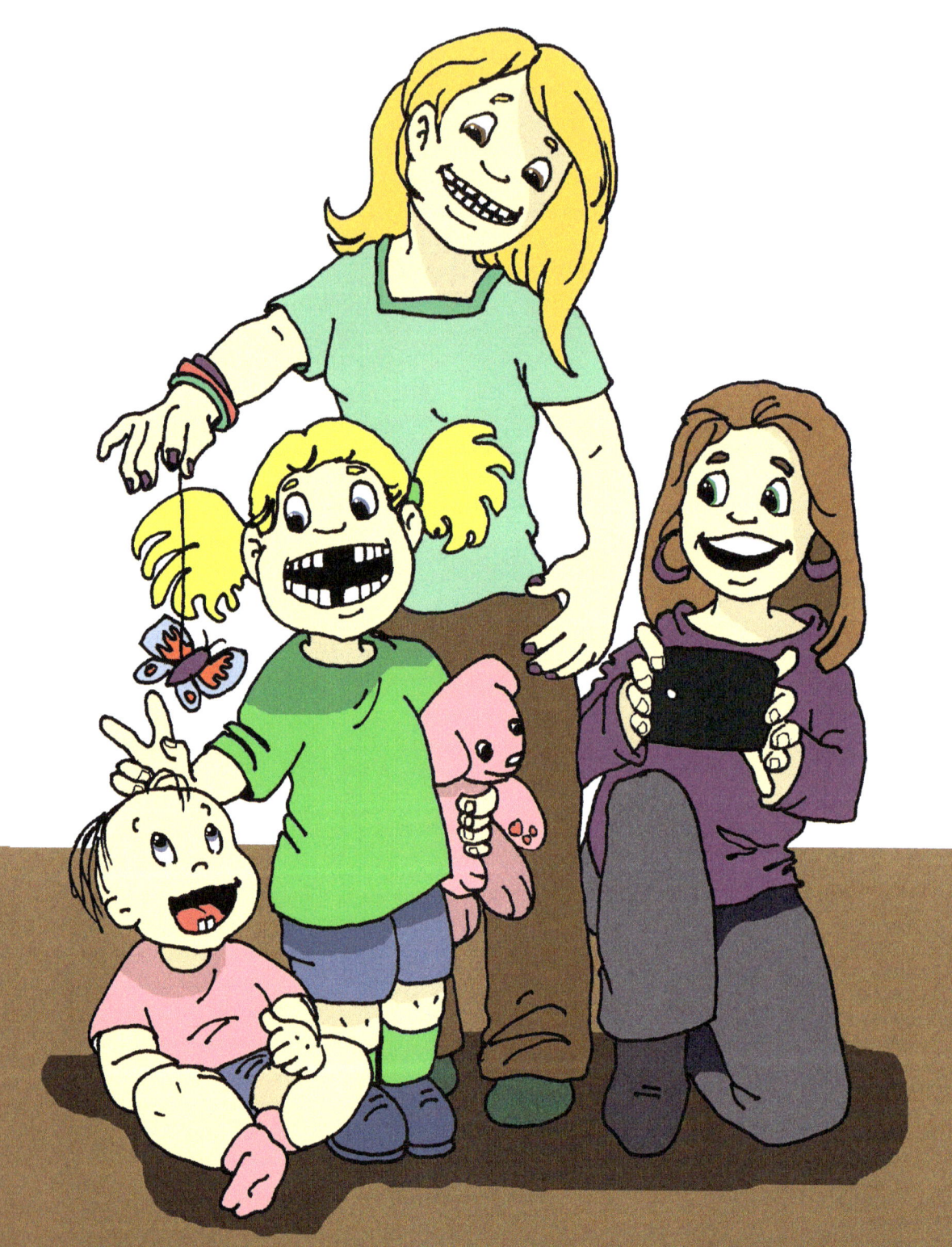

Tooth transitions. Pediatric Dentistry.

I have had the privilege to work with Dr. Charles Lekic at the Children's Hospital dental clinic. I have been working in the clinic since 1978. Dr. Lekic had a dream to make our clinic one of the most contemporary and functional hospital dental clinics in Canada. I never thought I would see it in my time working here. The clinic is beautiful. It was also his dream to start a graduate program in Pediatric Dentistry. So far, a total of six residents have graduated and become outstanding pediatric dentists. It is lucky for us that dreams do come true. Dr. Lekic is a very warm and dedicated pediatric dentist who loves to treat patients. He is an outstanding teacher who truly cares for his students and their success. His business savvy has been witnessed and appreciated. I have attended many meetings with Dr. Lekic over the years. He is so passionate to fight for what he believes in. In closing I would like to thank Dr. Lekic for everything he has done to make the Children's Hospital Dental Program a success and a pleasure to work in.

The attached cartoon illustrates the children that we care for. Infants to teens are a very fun group to work with. We are all very lucky to work with children. If you love what you do, you do not consider it work.

—Debbie Saunders

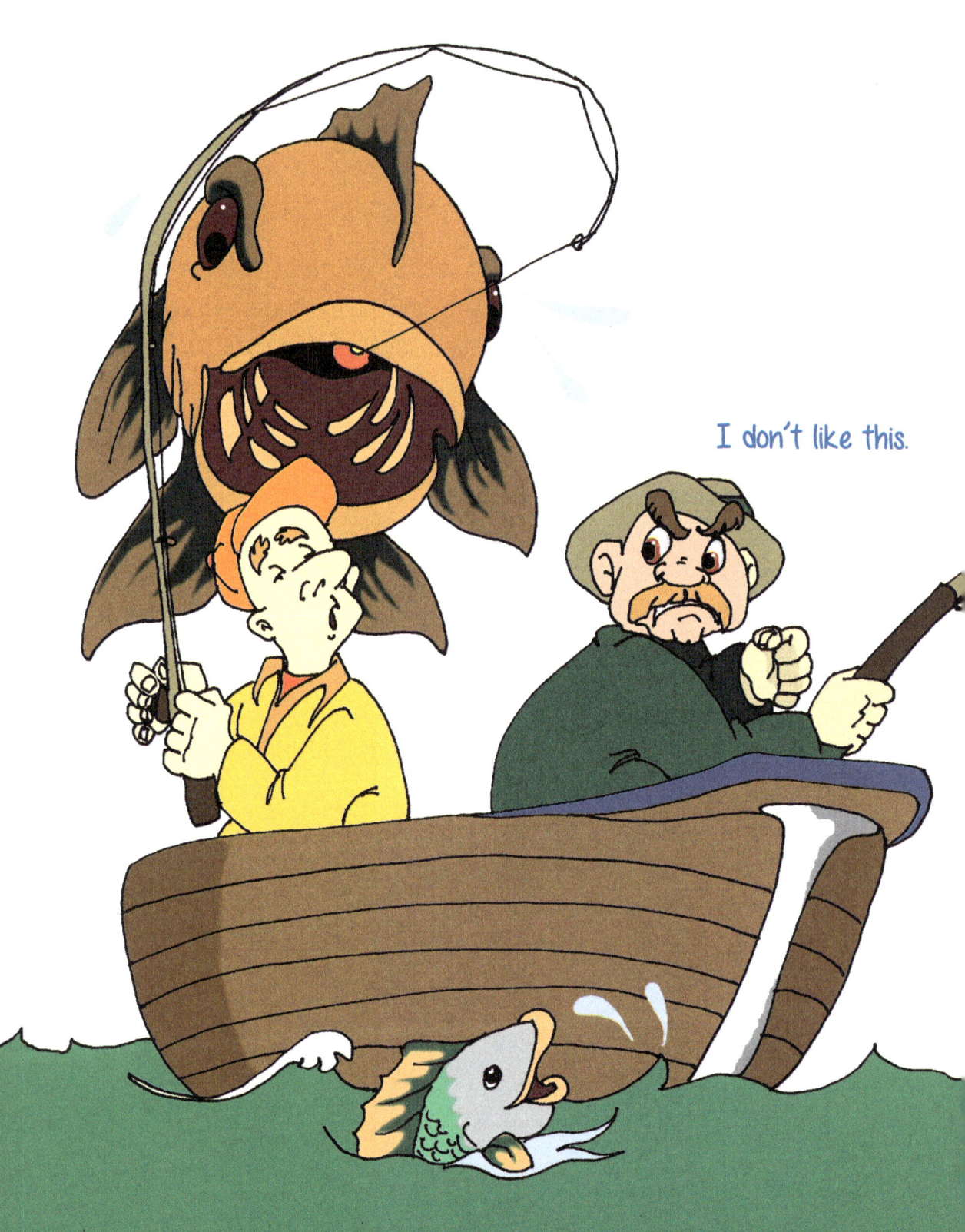

My favourite memories of Charles have very little to do with the academic realm or the College of Dentistry. Of course, this is the starting point for all my interactions with Charles, but he, more than any other person in my career, has demonstrated over and over again that true friendship and camaraderie can indeed start with a collegial working relationship. I will never forget three things that were enjoyable activities with Charles outside of the workplace (fishing, hockey games, and philosophical discourse over excellent single malt scotch or brandy).

Charles knew I liked fishing, and he made it a point to organize fishing trips even though he wasn't nearly as experienced in the finer points of catching fish. However, on one of the trips where we were fishing for sturgeon, he actually caught more than me. He noticed something wasn't quite right with my mood, and when I admitted to him I was a bit upset that he had "out-fished" me (something that no one had ever done before), he was overcome with laughter and told me he was not even paying attention to the number of fish caught. That is Charles, more concerned with someone else having a good time than the specifics of what is going on. We still joke about that fishing trip to this day.

Charles is a big hockey fan and frequently invited me to attend the Jets games in his family seats. Even though I was not a hockey fan, I always enjoyed attending with Charles and his family to witness their passion for the Jets. The outcome most nights was not favourable, and I enjoyed teasing Charles about how bad the Jets were compared to the New York and New Jersey teams that I grew up with during my time in the States. Charles was always a good sport about that, and each game always included a hearty break at the concession area for beer and hot dogs (always paid for by Charles of course). Everything I do know about hockey today is because of Charles.

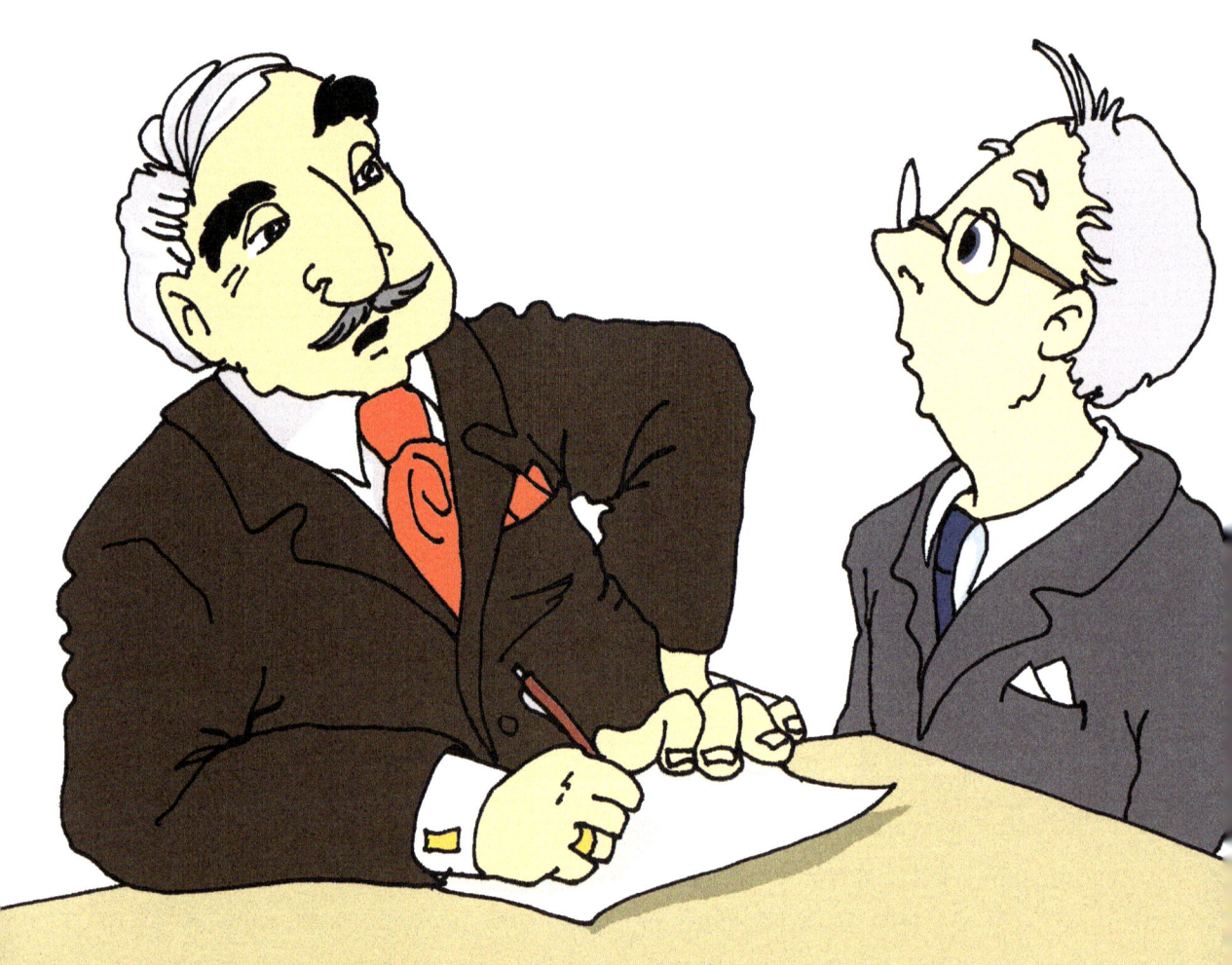

I have an offer that you won't want to refuse.

Charles knows quite a bit about the best single malt scotch (Lagavulin is one of his favourites) and brandy (Otard is the favourite here). We often met for dinner with our wives or were invited to his home for dinners, where he would pour these liberally and engage us in spirited philosophical discussions of the world, politics, and current events. This of course included movies and his favourite movie series of all time (*The Godfather*). There were so many times where we all repeated the famous lines of the movies and talked about how some of the characters and events were very similar to people and circumstances we encountered in our everyday lives in Winnipeg. It was always entertaining to hear the history of Charles and his family in the various places where they lived and also a pleasure to get to know each member of the Lekic family. There was no other place where you would feel so welcome.

—Tony Iacopino

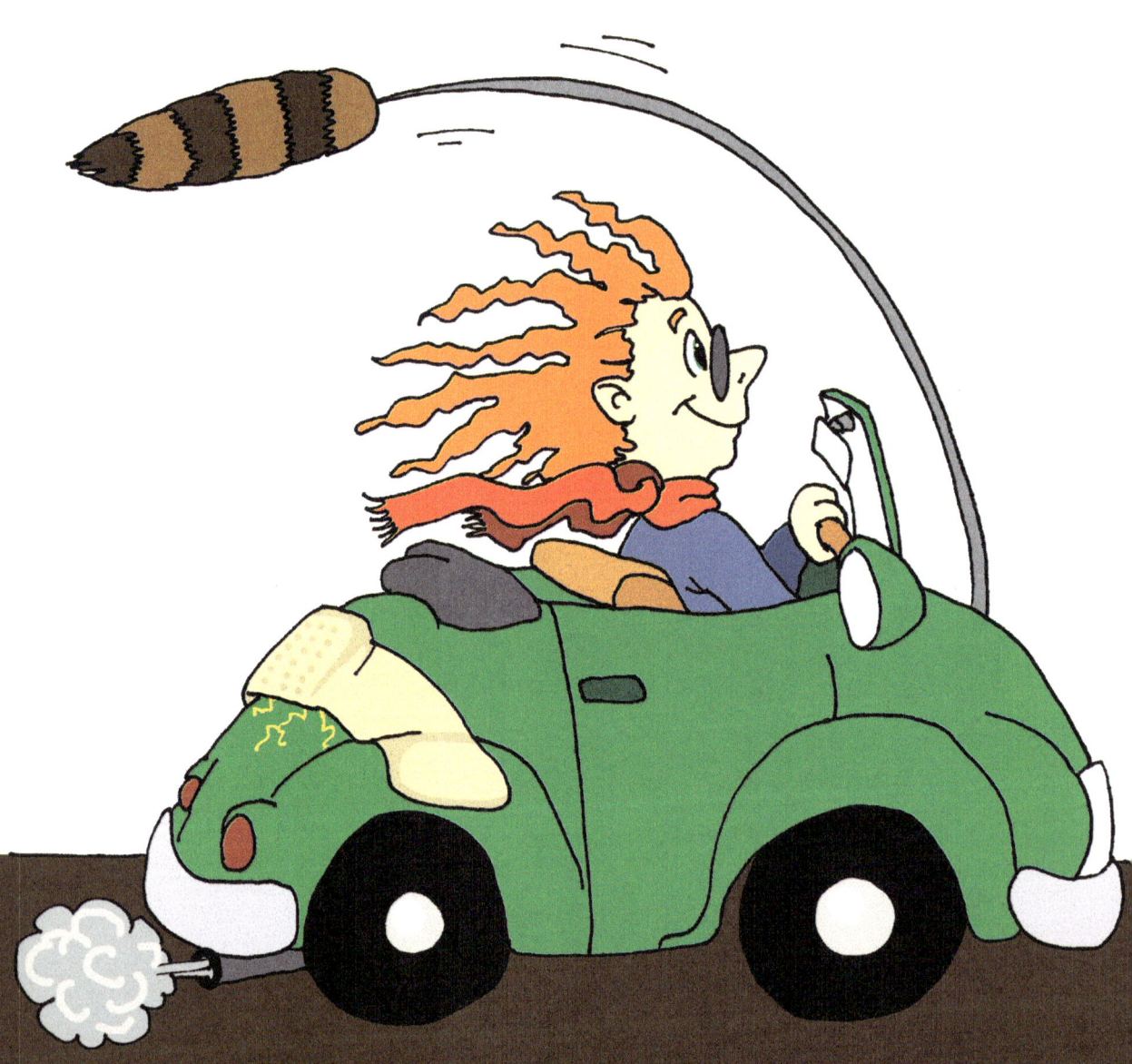

The happiest of people don't have the best of everything,
they just make the best of everything.

Working with between 10 and 20 years

Charles Lekic truly is the best boss that any person could have. He is considerate and makes time for you. I started working with Charles just over 16 years ago. He was a great boss and a friend. Often, he came in the office with a great cup of coffee for me. There is always fun happening in our area. On Halloween, Charles would dress up in costume for the children, and at Christmas time he was the jolliest Santa Claus, dressed in red and bringing gifts to all the children coming to the dental school for treatment. He was passionate at the projects he started, such as the Variety Children's Dental Outreach Program or the startup of the Graduate Program. I saw Charles first hand at being a kind and caring mentor, teacher, and advocate for all of his students. He would fight for any one of his students. On occasion, when we attended meetings off-site, I would have a ride in his beautiful, fast car. He has a definite love for cars and 70s music. Because of your charm and enthusiasm, regardless of it being hectic and crazy busy or just a regular day, Charles, I always had a smile coming to work, as I loved my job working with you and for you. Thank you, Charles, for making my position so rewarding and exciting that I looked forward to each day!

—Sandra Dufour
Pediatric Dentistry Office Staff

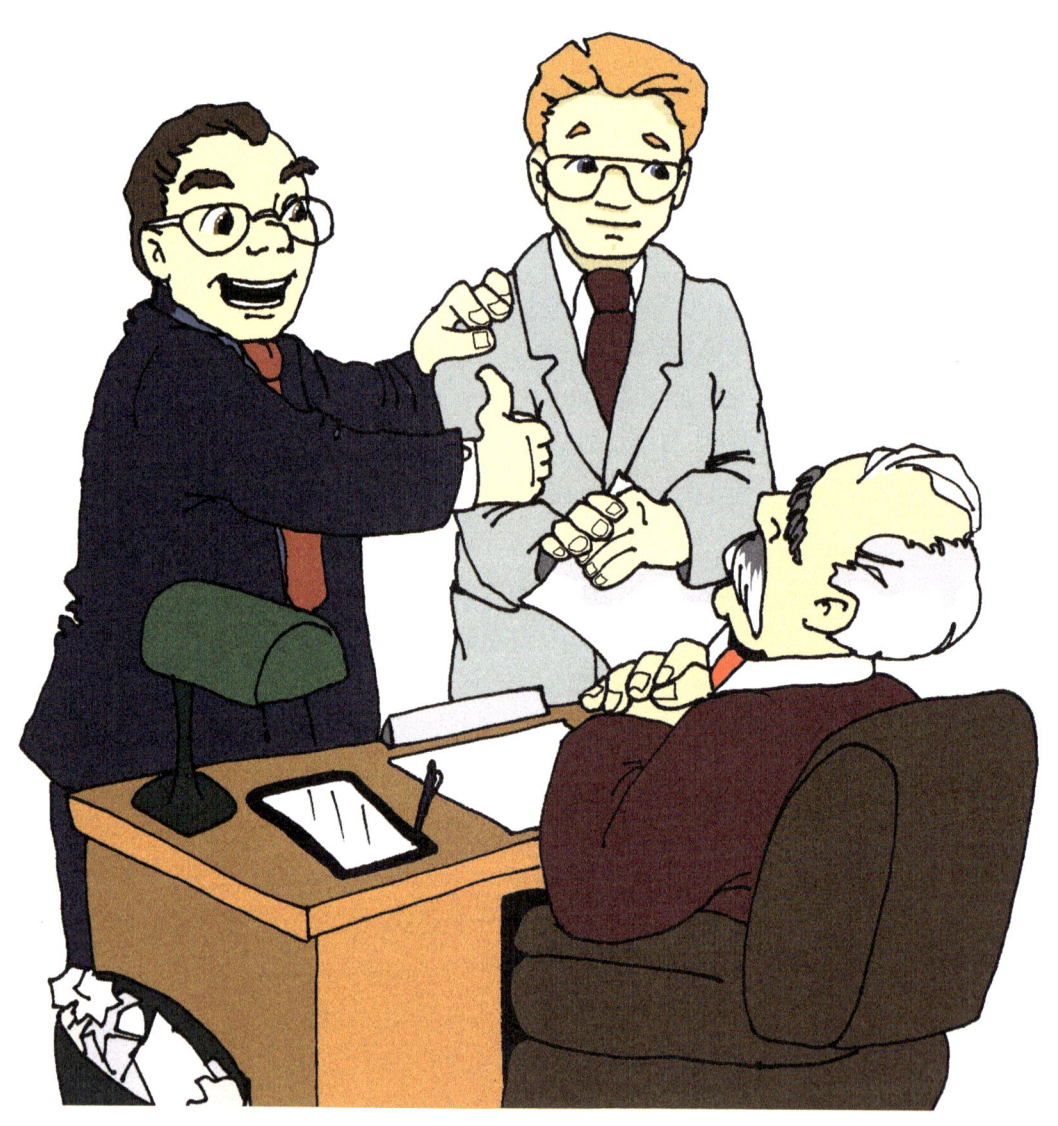

Look out for the people who look out for you.
Loyalty is everything.

To our dear friend, mentor and supervising dentist at the Grad Pedo Program.

It has been a wonderful experience to work with you at Children's Dental World; and when I left, it was with a pain in my heart that I did so. I went away for two years and was back working for you at the Grad Pedo program, doing your accounts receivable, and it was great working for and with you again.

You are one of the most loyal people I have met. We worked hard together to reach the goal that was set out to reach, and we did it!

I will miss you and know that you will be just as loyal and great to all the other people that cross your way in the future

Thank you for everything,
Leona Vos

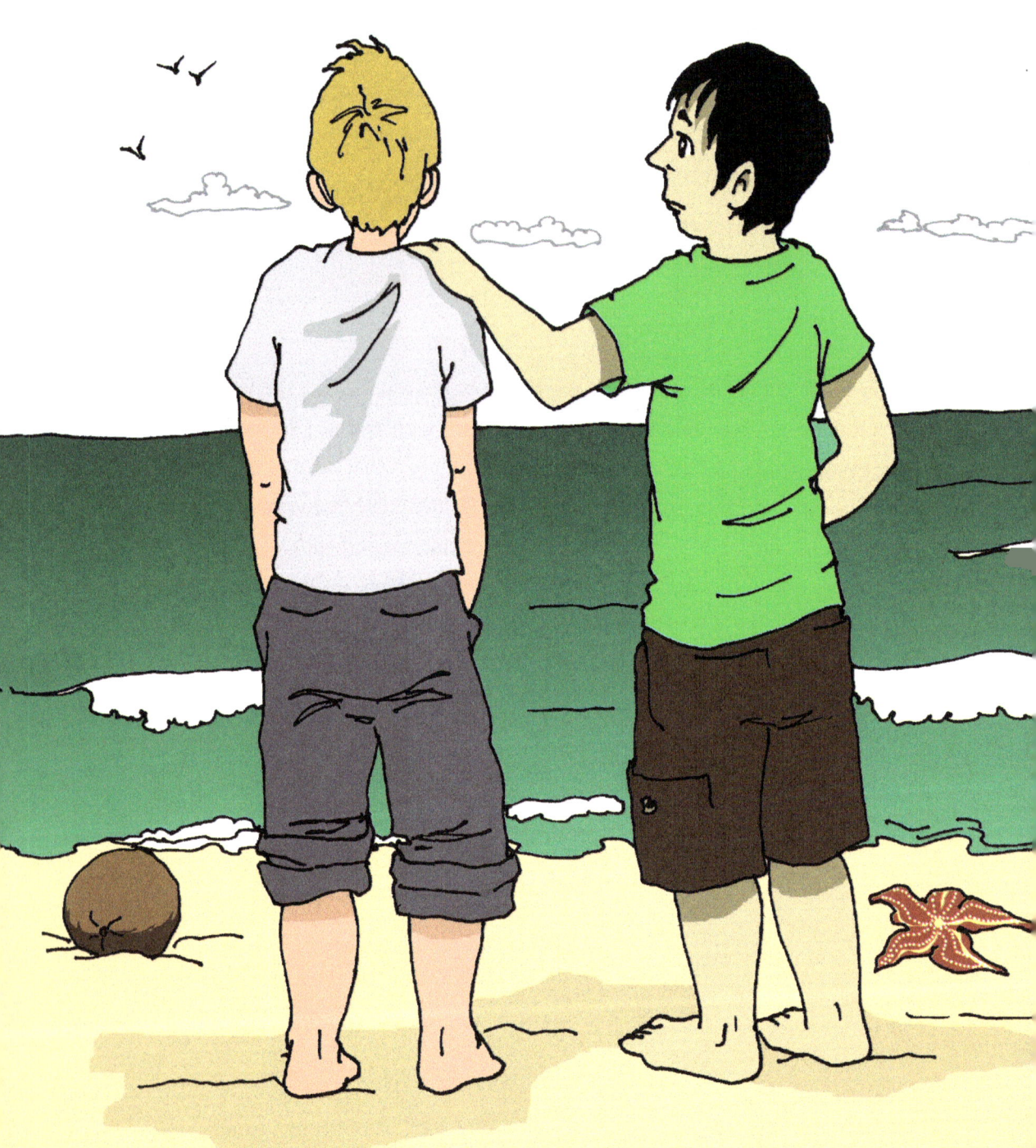

When you have been through hard times and come out the other side, look around you. The people still there are your true friends.

Working over 20 years

The first time I met Charles was just after he arrived in Winnipeg. Dr. Howard Cross was taking Charles around to meet all the Pediatric Dentists of the day. I had stepped away from teaching at the College the year before. Just after "hello," Charles said to me that he didn't care what the reason was for my leaving, he wanted me to return and that he would stand beside me.

At that time his support meant everything to me. We have stood by and supported each other from that day forward whenever necessary without either asking. "Brothers from different mothers!"

—Robert Diamond

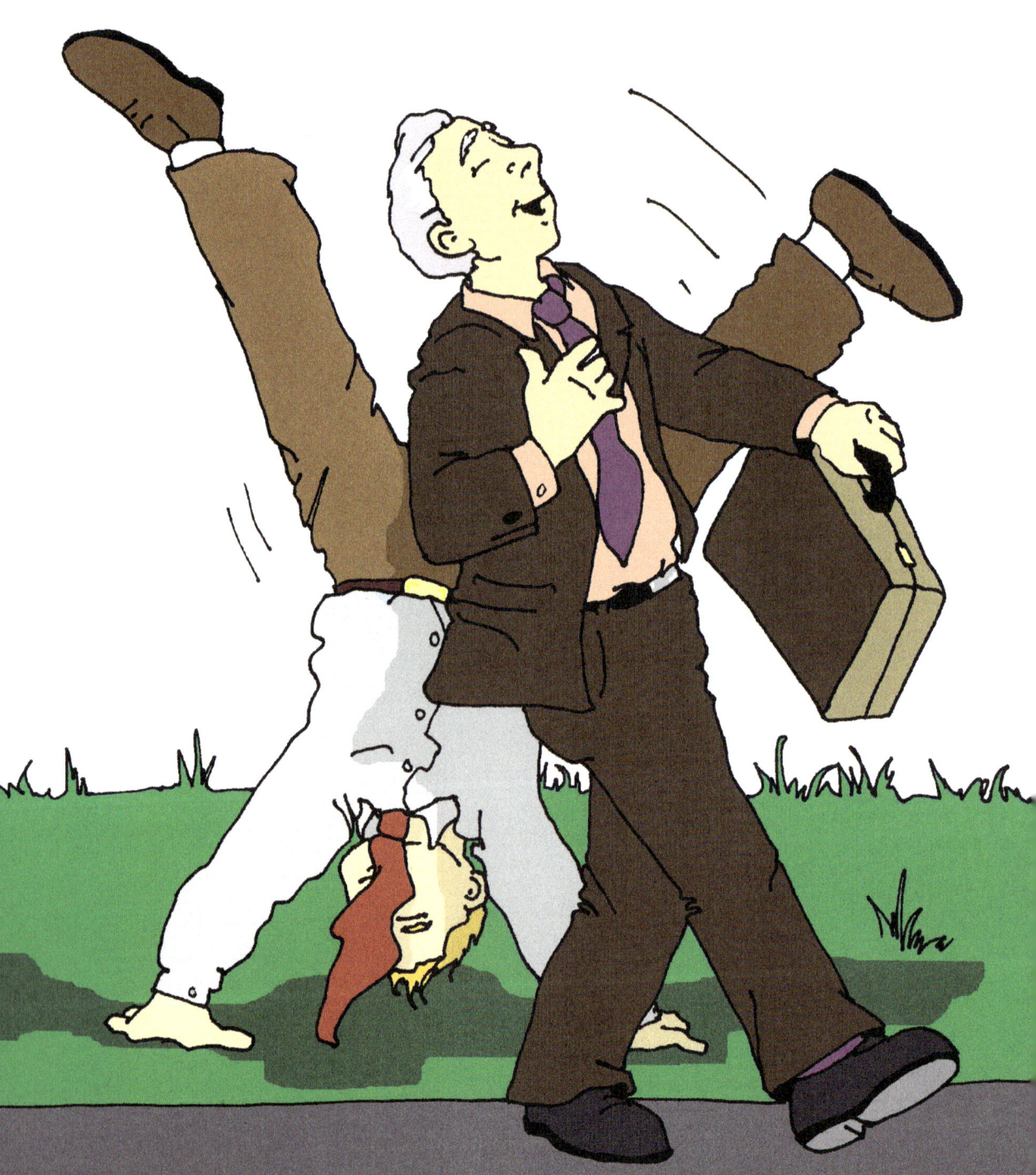

Best friends ... They know how crazy you are and still choose to be with you in public.

I was on the selection committee that interviewed Charles and offered him the job as Head of Undergraduate Pediatric Dentistry. Later, when he arrived to work, I picked him up at the airport and brought him home for a meal. He stayed overnight. We became instant friends. Charles and I used to go in the early morning to the track facility at the Medical College. We would jog several kilometres — we were younger then. We don't do this now (we know better).

I expect Charles, having been educated in Europe, to have an accent. However, on meeting him for the first time, I was surprised that he had none (well, perhaps a slight Transcona accent).

Charles and I liked to have breakfast at the Pancake House at 7:00 a.m. on Sunday mornings. We would discuss the state of Pediatric Dentistry, the university, and cars. Our wives thought we were crazy.

Charles and I both bought 2002 Ford Thunderbird convertibles – his black and mine red. He got speeding tickets – I didn't!

He wants a Tesla. Now, I suppose, I have to follow suit.

Charles and I bought Drones (more toys!).

Charles and I disagreed on the need for a Pediatric Dental Graduate Program. He was right.

Charles asked about the weather in Winnipeg. My response was that the weather was always exceptional. Exceptionally hot. Exceptionally cold. Exceptionally windy, exceptionally wet or snowy. He liked my explanation.

Charles is a talker. At dinner Charles will talk while we eat. He eats his dinner after we have finished. His stories are always fascinating, but hunger trumps fascination.

Charles likes to drive fast. He had collected several tickets for speeding and was on probation. Recently, he was stopped for ignoring a school zone – unwittingly (really). He produced his Saskatchewan driver's licence, and the cop gave him a warning as an out of towner. (What luck!)

—Howard Cross

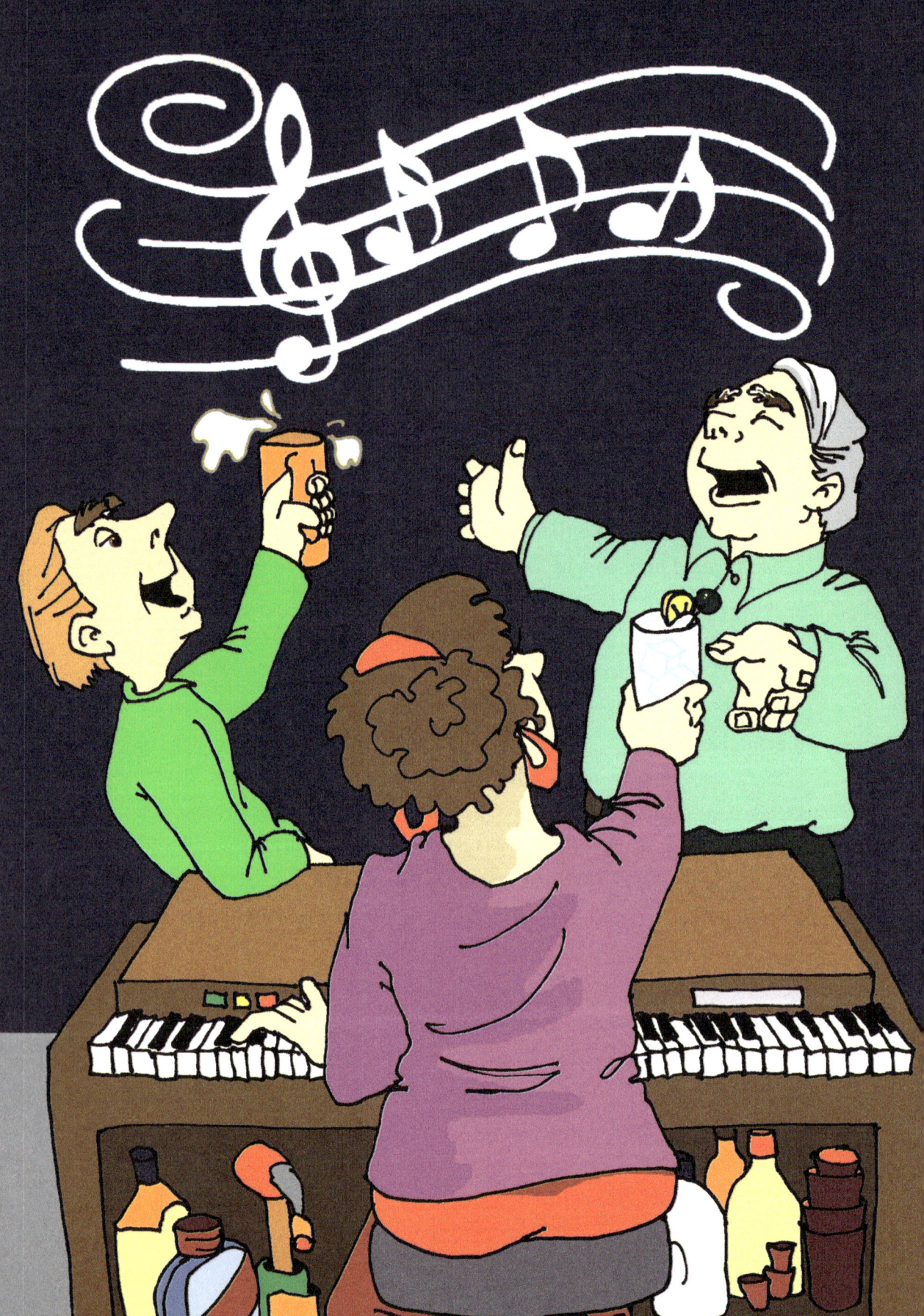

My personal "Charles story"

We met 20 years ago in 1996, having both been appointed within a few months of each other as Head of "Pedo" and Head of "Ortho", respectively. Charles arrived about three months ahead of me, at the start of a Winnipeg winter, via Toronto from the former Republic of Yugoslavia, and I from South Africa. Needless to say, we both found Winnipeg to be a very cold place, and is still today, with flurries on the 13th May, maybe because today is Friday the 13th! The year we met in 1996 still holds the record for the coldest in history, with the most number of continuous days below freezing on record, and that was followed by the April 1997 Flood of the Century!

Charles and I would look out the window of our offices together and say, "What are we doing here – are we crazy?" But with emotional support from each other, we remained positive, and survived, while people were saying, "Oh, they won't be here for long, and they will move somewhere warm" – well, Charles – we proved them wrong – 20 years hence and we are still here, just much thicker skinned in more ways than one!

In those early days, Zivka, Milos, and Nick were still living in Toronto, and Charles and I in downtown Winnipeg, near each other in high rise apartment blocks and since Charles and I needed to eat a good meal from time to time, we tried out just about every restaurant in Winnipeg and often ended up at the piano bar here at the Fort Garry Hotel on a Friday night, when Charles didn't go back to Toronto to visit his family. Needless to say, we spent a fortune at the Piano Bar on single malt whiskeys and cognac during the first six months of our new lives in Winnipeg. One day at the piano bar, Charles told me he was so lonely without his family here that we went to the pet shelter and got him a cat named Bloo to keep him company. I guess he named him Bloo to keep away the winter blues sans his family at his side during those first months in Winterpeg, Manisnowba!

And that is how Charles and I survived our first winter in Winnipeg, our great friendship with each other, trying out every Winnipeg restaurant, meeting up at the piano bar, drinking single malt whiskey, cognac, and the company of Charles' cat, Bloo!

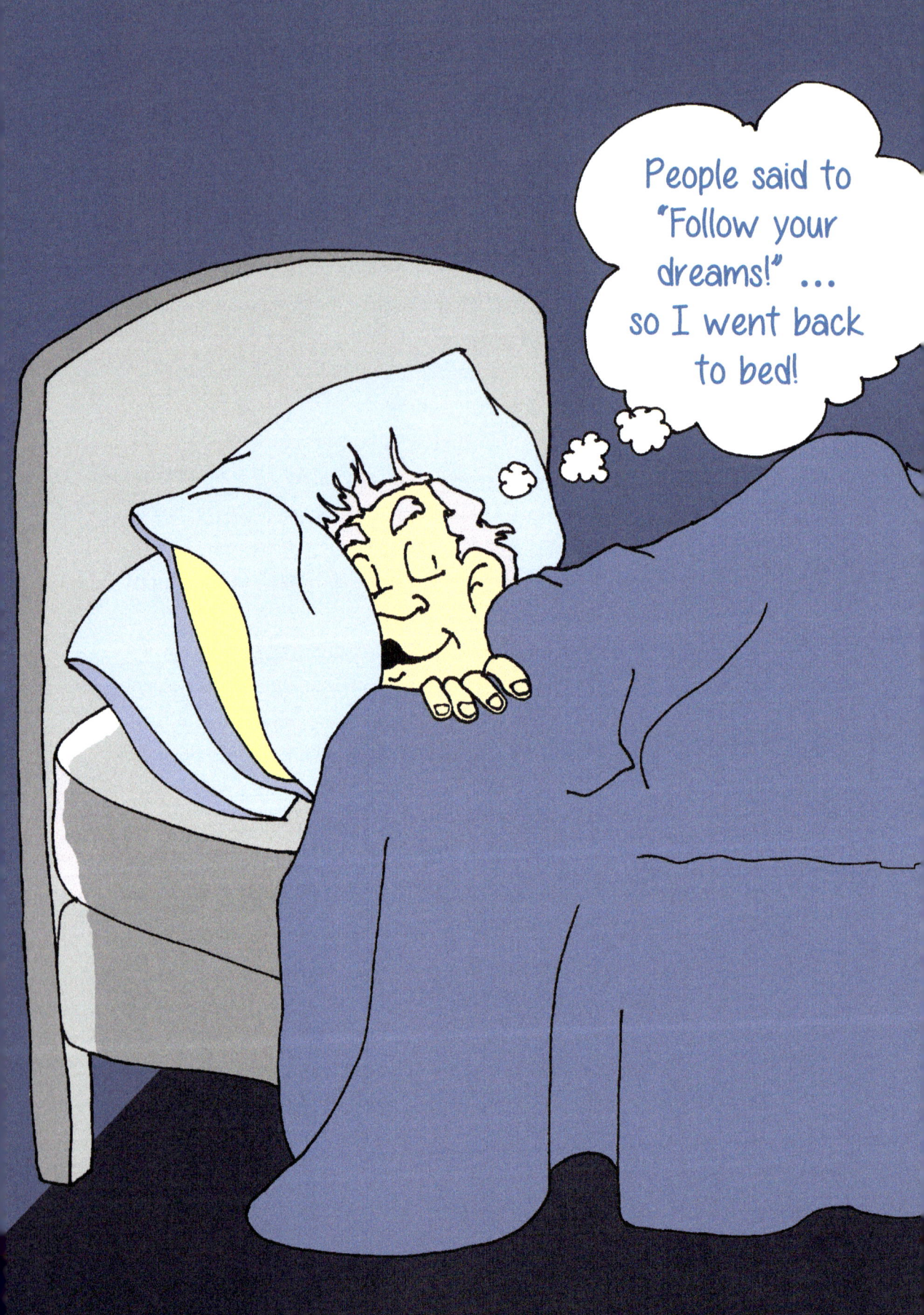

Before we arrived in Winnipeg, due to budget cuts at the time (Remember those Filman Fridays?) and staff shortages in both pedo and ortho (nothing's changed in 20 years ... right), the faculty voted to merge PDS and DDSS into one mega-department, named DDSS. From our first few months together here at the university, Charles and I had a dream to re-establish the PDS department. With the strong support of the late and great Dr. David Singer, department head at the time, and Doug Brothwell, who had just been appointed as head of Community Dentistry, we began a long uphill battle starting in 1998, against all odds and with much resistance, to re-establish the Department of Preventive Dental Science. One of the major visions and dreams of the envisaged new department, way back in 1998, was to establish a new Pediatric Dentistry Graduate Program. And of course, Charles championed this dream and kept the dream alive, never giving up.

Finally, in 2001, Faculty Council and Senate approval laid the foundation stones for the re-birth of PDS. And hence began the next uphill battle – to establish a Pediatric Dentistry residency program in PDS. Despite opposition from many, we did eventually realize Charles' dream in 2011 – thirteen years after Charles advocated to make this an important goal for a newly established PDS. And so, as a result of Charles' ongoing tenacity, this proud year in 2016, the third group of Pedo residents, will graduate from the program, making up the first six program alumni and the fifth great anniversary year of the PDGP. This program is there only because Charles dreamed about it, was willing to continue to fight for it, and never gave up – despite all the odds and due to his enduring tenacity. In fact, I have told Charles on many occasions that he is the most tenacious person I know. When the university and COPSE and the provincial government approved the progam, they did so without any financial involvement – but even that didn't stop Charles. What did he do? He went and took a $1.3 million loan, which he paid off in a record time of only two years. And that, ladies and gentlemen, is the calibre of the man that Charles is, the man we are honouring here tonight.

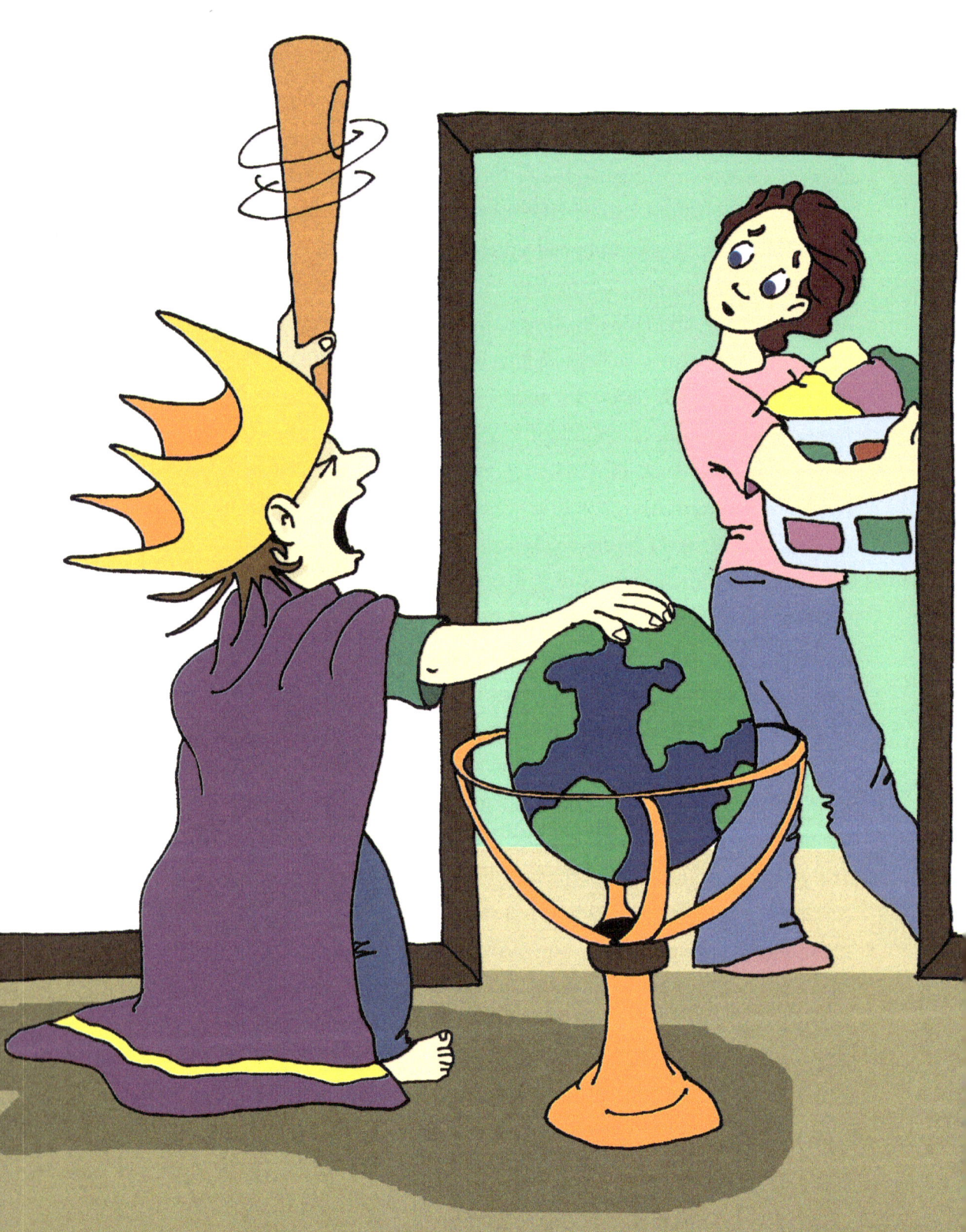
I got plans, BIG PLANS, I say!

But wait, there is more – the program got accredited right out of its starting gates, and all its residents who have taken the RCDC and American Boards have passed at their first effort. What a phenomenal accolade for a new program and its remarkable program director.

What Charles accomplished here reminds me of the words of the great American architect Daniel Burnham, who said and I quote: "Make no little plans; they have no magic to stir men's blood and probably themselves will not be realized. Make big plans; aim high in hope and work, remembering that a noble, logical plan once recorded will never die, but long after we are gone be a living thing, asserting itself with ever-growing insistency."

Charles' legacy to this university is the PDGP, which I know will continue to assert itself with ever-growing insistency into the future.

Personally, I know Charles as a kind and generous man, one of fairness, honesty, loyalty, and integrity, a strong student advocate and someone who is willing to fight for what is right and good, and so it came to be that Charles and I challenged the bylaws of the MDA to ensure that dental professionals emigrating to Canada could also have a rightful place in the sun in this great country of ours – Canada. Again, against all odds and with few friends at our side other than the great Dr. David Singer, we spent three years fighting to ensure that there would be a pathway for internationally trained dentists to become fully licensed in Canada; and together with a group in Newfoundland, we caused the regulatory authorities across Canada to institute a fair and non-discriminatory system of licensing and registration.

So, I hope by now, ladies and gentlemen, you are able to see just why I call Charles "my brother from another mother", for together we have crossed many miles, carrying each other across fields lain with landmines and seas strewn with icebergs, in our path to success. Ladies and gentlemen, indeed, Charles as a person personifies to me the words of Sir Edmund Hillary of Everest fame, and I quote: *"If the going is tough and the pressure is on; if reserves of strength have been drained and the summit is still not in sight; then the quality to seek in a man is neither great strength nor quickness of hand, but rather a resolute mind firmly set on its purpose that refuses to let its body slacken or rest."*

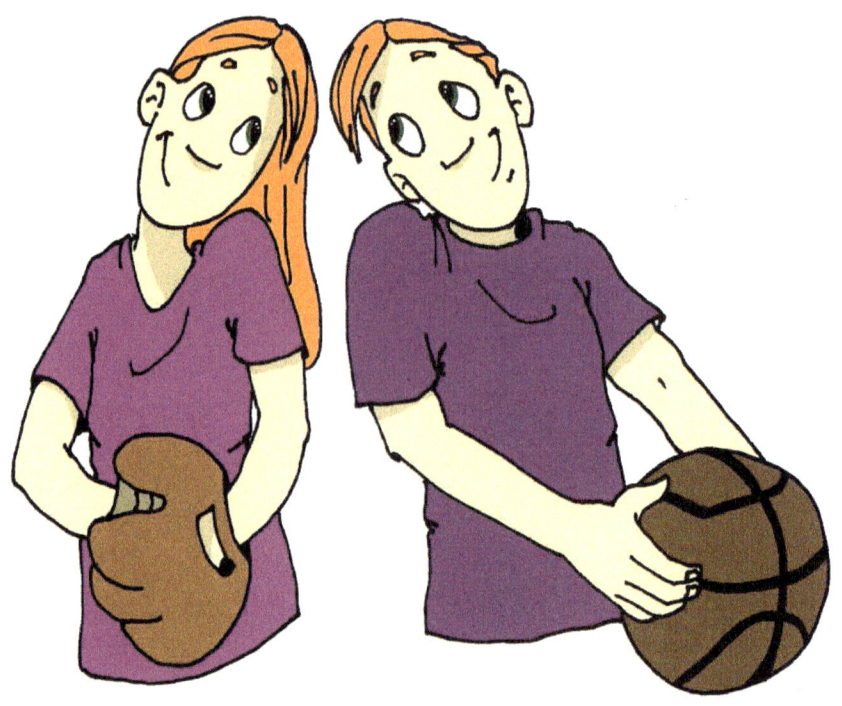

A true friend is the brother or sister you never had, yet you adopt them as family from another Mother.

Charles, my friend, my academic brother, while I wish you a happy retirement from the university, it is with much sadness that I see you leave, for together we fought many good fights and what we achieved we did through each other's strong support, strong respect, love of our work, respect for our students, and many late-night phone calls, often lasting for hours, to solve the problems that sought to trip us up.

The success of 15 years of our PDS department has been a team effort, and you have played a vital leadership role as Division Head of PD in making it a success story through your valiant efforts with Variety and the Bussing Program and ensuring our undergraduate program in PD remains one of the brightest jewels in the PDS crown.

Charles, you have been fortunate to have enjoyed the support and love of your family who are here with us tonight, and I would like to thank and acknowledge Zivka, Milos, and Nick for their love and support of you in your academic role at the university and the important parts they played during the past 20 years while you gave your all and dedicated your time unselfishly to the University of Manitoba.

Charles, in closing, allow me to share these final words with you, which I came across on the coffee table while visiting my mother recently; they are appropriate for you and personify you. It is by an unknown author and is entitled "Greatness," and I quote:

A man is as great as the dreams he dreams
As great as the love he bears
As great as the values he redeems
As the happiness he shares

A man is as great as the thoughts he thinks
As the worth he has attained
As the fountains at which his spirit drinks
As the insight he has gained

A man is as great as the truth he speaks
As great as the help he gives
As great as the destiny he seeks
He is indeed as great as the life he lives

Charles, there is no doubt in my mind that you are living a great life, the life you carved out for yourself; one can say you have lived and continue to live your dream; so, my friend, my good friend, my brother, I salute you, I thank you, I will miss you and our runs to go and get coffee. May God continue to bless you.

Thank you
BILLY WILTSHIRE

Summary

Shared in the pages of this book are memories and experiences as remembered and written by my former students and staff members. I was touched deeply reading these words. The text was sent back to each contributor for their review and changed prior to publishing; however, the returned text remained essentially unchanged. As emotions settled, I realized that the 44 individuals who contributed have addressed a number of positive issues. Of course, it is possible that others who may have had a different point of view decided not to send their comments. Nevertheless, it could be argued that even if only one life was touched, then my life may have been worth dreaming and living.

Overall, the excitement of academic life is not related to the salary line, as working in private dental practice, income may be three to four times higher. The faculty meetings are not much better, as often they are lengthy in time and low in accomplishment, rarely achieving results beyond the starting point. Similar are the university rules since they would rarely promote financial incentives and individual successes followed with achieving increase revenue, but would often result in supporting others who have been unsuccessful! Is what is said inviting enough to take on an academic dental position? Probably not. However, viewing the memories and the experiences of our graduates and staff members raise another issue that should be considered.

The graduates that responded described the care they received as an important attribute in helping them through their studies and in preparing them well to serve within the dental profession. How valuable was this and can it ever be measured through financial remuneration, hours spent at faculty meetings, or adherence to the university rules? In the author's mind and heart, the answer is NO. Nothing can be as important as touching the lives of others and, in doing so, making a difference in them. This is something far beyond personal gains or feelings, and knowing that after many years the work left behind is still valued and appreciated is priceless.

The dream that is over 30 years old lives on and invites and challenges members of our profession to consider making a difference in the lives of others by embracing the academic life.

Will you regret it? I am sure I never did.

Thank you

P.S. These beautiful drawings are the work of an amazing illustrator from Denver Colorado, Shannon Parish (www.shannonparish.com).

Thank you Shannon

CPSIA information can be obtained
at www.ICGtesting.com
Printed in the USA
LVOW05s1715051117
555054LV00001B/1/P

9 781525 516528